LUPUS

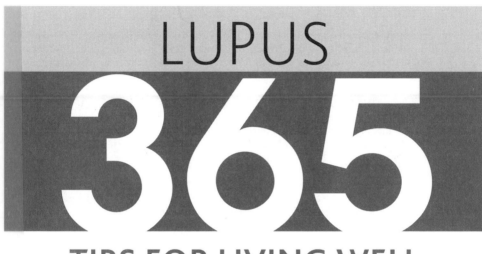

LUPUS
365
TIPS FOR LIVING WELL

Jessica Rowshandel, LMSW

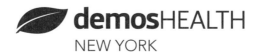

demosHEALTH
NEW YORK

Visit our website at www.demoshealth.com

ISBN: 978-1-936303-87-8
e-book ISBN: 978-1-61705-251-4

Acquisitions Editor: Julia Pastore
Compositor: diacriTech

Medical information provided by Demos Health, in the absence of a visit with a health care professional, must be considered as an educational service only. This book is not designed to replace a physician's independent judgment about the appropriateness or risks of a procedure or therapy for a given patient. Our purpose is to provide you with information that will help you make your own health care decisions.

The information and opinions provided here are believed to be accurate and sound, based on the best judgment available to the authors, editors, and publisher, but readers who fail to consult appropriate health authorities assume the risk of injuries. The publisher is not responsible for errors or omissions. The editors and publisher welcome any reader to report to the publisher any discrepancies or inaccuracies noticed.

Library of Congress Cataloging-in-Publication Data
Rowshandel, Jessica.
 Lupus : 365 tips for living well / Jessica Rowshandel, LMSW.
   pages cm
 Includes bibliographical references and index.
 ISBN 978-1-936303-87-8 — ISBN 978-1-61705-251-4 (e-book)
 1. Systemic lupus erythematosus—Popular works. 2. Systemic lupus erythematosus—Treatment—Popular works. I. Title.
 RC924.5.L85R69 2015
 616.7'72—dc23
                                    2015036143

Special discounts on bulk quantities of Demos Health books are available to corporations, professional associations, pharmaceutical companies, health care organizations, and other qualifying groups. For details, please contact:

Special Sales Department
Demos Health
11 West 42nd Street, 15th Floor
New York, NY 10036
Phone: 800-532-8663 or 212-683-0072
Fax: 212-941-7842
E-mail: specialsales@springerpub.com

Printed in the United States of America by McNaughton & Gunn.
15 16 17 18 19 / 5 4 3 2 1

For the members of my lupus support group, with gratitude

Contents

Introduction   xi

Part I: The Basics

1. Understanding Lupus   3

2. Getting the Medical Care You Need   9

Find a Lupus Doctor   9

If You are Underinsured or Uninsured   13

Prescription Assistance   16

Preparing for Your First Visit   17

Communicating with Your Doctor   19

3. Medication and Treatment   23

Manage Your Medication   23

Complementary and Alternative Treatment   27

Real versus Fake Science   32

Part II: Living Well

4. You Are Not Alone   39

Find Support   39

Lupus and Grief   41

Lupus and Depression   42

5. Men with Lupus   45

6. Maintaining a Healthy Lifestyle   47

Lupus and Nutrition   47

Strive for a Healthy Lifestyle   49

7. Managing Stress   53

Plan Ahead for a Flare   53

Manage Energy Levels   56

More Stress Management Tools   58

8. Managing Lupus Fog   61

9. Lupus on the Outside   65

Part III: Lupus and Personal Relationships

10. Family and Friends   71

Support from Friends and Family   71

Maintaining a Social Life   75

Managing Busy Holidays   76

11. Romantic Relationships   79

Dating   79

Sex   81

Family Planning   83

12. Parenting   87

Part IV: Navigating the World with Lupus

13. Advance Directives   93

14. Work   97

15. Disability Benefits   101

16. Higher Education   107

17. Traveling   111

18. Becoming a Lupus Advocate   115

Create Lupus Awareness   115

Advocate for Health Care Policy and Funding   117

Help Make Medicine More Patient Centered   118

Clinical Trials   119

Afterword   121

Resources   123

Acknowledgments   133

Index   135

Introduction

Sometimes it might feel as if lupus has taken over your life. That's because lupus impacts every part of it, the most obvious being your physical health. If you don't feel well, it's hard to live the life you're used to or the one you had planned. Lupus can impact your self-esteem and emotional health, social life, romantic relationships, family life, ability to work, income, and personal goals. It can feel overwhelming and bleak. This is why it's important to have the tools to manage these parts of your life and reduce the impact lupus has on them. In turn, you will improve your quality of life. This book is filled with hundreds of tips to help you do that.

With this book, you will learn how to obtain medical care, which is step one. You will then learn how to become an active participant in your health care and how to advocate for yourself in many areas of your life. The book ends with tips on how to get involved with awareness and advocacy activities in the lupus community. There are also resources in the back, including contact information and website addresses. These will help you learn more about topics covered in some chapters and connect with relevant organizations.

The book's structure reflects how learning to live well with lupus builds on itself—from the important foundations of learning about lupus and obtaining medical care, to addressing specific personal needs, to broad community issues. When developing this structure, I was inspired by the proverb, "Little by little, a little becomes a lot." The proverb is also a reminder that progress does not happen overnight and does not need to happen fast. With the hundreds of tips in this book, if you take on too many at once you will feel tired and overwhelmed. Start small and with what's most important to you, and build on them little by little.

Don't strive for perfection. Perfection is impossible, and striving for it creates a lot of pressure and disappointment. Do the best you can for where you are in life today. Some days that will mean doing less. Sometimes you will do more. Go at your own pace. Be patient and compassionate with yourself. Remind yourself that you are doing the best you can.

As the former Director of Social Services of the S.L.E. Lupus Foundation, I listened to the stories of hundreds of people with lupus who all did their best. At support groups, they showed each other the compassion that they sometimes had trouble showing themselves. Sometimes we have trouble taking our own advice, and we need the help of others. I facilitated the groups, but even I found myself in this situation. If I hadn't listened to the stories of my support group members, I would have never seen a rheumatologist for my lifelong, but worsening, symptoms of body pain and fatigue. I was finally diagnosed with fibromyalgia. With this diagnosis, I suddenly had a fresh understanding of many of the coping strategies we spoke about at length in the groups.

Though there are some similar symptoms, lupus is not fibromyalgia, and it was only through these stories that I gained a better understanding of what life with lupus is like. In order to translate lupus from a list of symptoms to a real experience, we need these stories. But even more important is that I got to know who each group member was and learned, first hand, that no matter what, lupus does not define anyone no matter how much it feels like lupus has taken over. You are not lupus. You are much more than lupus, and hopefully this book will help you continue to realize and live that.

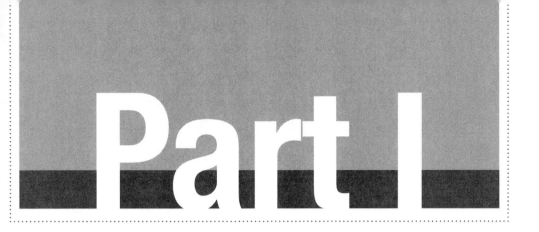

The Basics

Understanding Lupus

Having a basic understanding of lupus will help you feel more in control over managing the disease. It will also help you understand the importance of treatment and making lifestyle changes that will improve your quality of life. The more you know about lupus, the more you can communicate with your doctor about changes in symptoms and concerns or questions you might have. You are your best advocate. I always remind people, "Knowledge is power," so the more you know about how this disease could impact your body, the more empowered you could feel to monitor it and do the best you can to manage it.

Systemic Lupus Erythematosus

Systemic Lupus Erythematosus (SLE, or lupus for short) is a chronic autoimmune disease that can affect any part of the body including the skin, joints, muscles, kidneys, heart and cardiovascular system, lungs, and the brain and central nervous system. Most people with lupus experience fatigue and pain in the muscles and joints. No two people with lupus have the same combination of symptoms. Lupus is also a disease of periods, called flares, when symptoms increase, and periods when symptoms improve.

What Is an Autoimmune Disease?

Having an autoimmune disease means that a person has an overactive immune system. Healthy immune systems send proteins called antibodies to attack foreign invaders like viruses and other germs that cause infection. But when someone has an autoimmune disease, their immune system gets confused and sends auto- (self) antibodies to attack that person's own body and healthy tissue. It is acting in overdrive, attacking "germs" that are not really there.

Different autoimmune diseases are associated with different parts of the body. For example, type 1 diabetes causes a person's immune system to attack the pancreas. Lupus is systemic, meaning any part of the body can be affected.

Lupus Is Not...

Lupus is not a sexually transmitted disease. It is not contagious. It is not spread by a virus or bacteria. It is not cancer. It is not a blood disorder.

The Cause and Cure Are Unknown

What causes lupus to develop is not well understood, and there is no cure. There is medication, however, that can help people manage the disease. Lupus is a chronic condition, which means that people manage it for the rest of their lives. Lupus treatment has improved over the last several decades and now, with better treatment, people with lupus can live a normal life span.

Who Develops Lupus?

It is estimated that about 1.5 million people in the United States have lupus. Anyone of any age, gender, race, or ethnicity can develop lupus, including children, males, and older adults. But about nine out of ten people who develop lupus are female; the typical age of onset is 15 to 45 years old, and African Americans, Latinos, Native Americans, and Asians are two to three times more likely than Caucasians to develop it.

Skin Lupus

The second most common type of lupus is cutaneous lupus erythematosus, also referred to as skin lupus. There are three categories of skin lupus: chronic cutaneous lupus (CCLE), subacute cutaneous lupus (SCLE), and acute cutaneous lupus (ACLE). Discoid lupus erythematosus (DLE) is one type of CCLE, and is a common type of skin lupus.

Skin lupus symptoms can include hair loss; changes in the pigment of the skin; sensitivity to UV rays from the sun or artificial light; mouth, nasal, or genital sores; rashes and lesions that can be red, scaly, and/or itchy and can sometimes lead to scarring; and other skin-related symptoms. The malar or "butterfly" rash, often mistaken for rosacea or sunburn, is a symptom of both skin lupus and SLE.

While people with SLE can exhibit these skin symptoms, skin lupus does not affect other systems of the body or involve joint and muscle pain and fatigue. Yet, it can drastically alter a person's appearance, causing emotional and psychological distress.

Most people who have skin lupus — about 90% — do not develop SLE. If you suspect skin lupus, you should see a dermatologist, preferably one with experience with lupus or autoimmune diseases.

Neonatal Lupus

If a mother has certain lupus-related antibodies called anti-Ro and anti-La, they can cause symptoms of neonatal lupus in the baby. Neonatal lupus is not the infant form of lupus. It is a rare condition in newborns who temporarily experience lupus symptoms such as skin rashes and liver and blood problems. These symptoms typically disappear after six months with no lasting effects. Another symptom of neonatal lupus is congenital heart block, a slow heart rhythm that, depending on severity, might need to be treated with a pacemaker.

Drug-Induced Lupus

Drug-induced lupus is not a true form of lupus and is rare. Certain types of medication used to treat high blood pressure, seizures, tuberculosis, and several other conditions can cause lupus-like symptoms. In this case, the immune system is overreacting to the medication. Symptoms go away after the medication is stopped. People experiencing lupus-like symptoms must tell their doctor right away so they can be safely taken off the medication.

What Is a Rheumatologist?

A rheumatologist is a medical doctor (MD) or doctor of osteopathic medicine (DO) who specializes in treating rheumatic diseases. These diseases of the musculoskeletal system affect the bones, joints, muscles, and connective tissue like ligaments, tendons, and cartilage. Examples of rheumatic diseases include arthritis, Sjögren's syndrome, myositis, scleroderma, and SLE. It is important to choose a rheumatologist with experience treating lupus.

Trouble Getting a Diagnosis

Many people go to several doctors before they get a diagnosis. Lupus symptoms can seem vague and hard to pinpoint or can be confused with other conditions. A doctor might hear that a person is tired and think that this is due to stress. They might think body pain is due to arthritis, or that a fever is due to a virus. This is why lupus is sometimes referred to as the "Great Imitator." Some patients are told that their symptoms are "all in their head." For these reasons, a lupus diagnosis is often missed.

Diagnosing Lupus

There is no one lupus test that will tell you if you have lupus. If you suspect that you have lupus, you should see a rheumatologist. The rheumatologist will ask you about your medical history, your symptoms, and your family medical history; conduct a complete physical exam; and take blood for a complete blood count and antibody blood tests (e.g., ANA, anti-dsDNA, anti-Sm) that could help determine if you have lupus. Your rheumatologist will also obtain a urine sample to check how your kidneys are functioning.

The American College of Rheumatology created a list of 11 criteria of lupus symptoms. These criteria are categories of symptoms that were created for research purposes. In order to do lupus research, lupus has to be clearly defined, and people need to meet at least four of these criteria to be given a lupus diagnosis. However, outside of research, lupus can be strongly suspected or diagnosed with less than four of these symptoms.

The American College of Rheumatology's 11 Criteria

1. **Malar rash**—A butterfly-shaped rash across the cheeks and the bridge of the nose, one "wing" on each cheek.
2. **Discoid rash**—A rash that is raised, red, and scaly. Patches can be oval or round.
3. **Photosensitivity**—People with lupus can be sensitive to sunlight or fluorescent lights. The sensitivity is to the UVA and UVB rays, which can trigger lupus symptoms.
4. **Mouth or nose ulcers**—However, not all ulcers are lupus related.
5. **Nonerosive arthritis**—Nonerosive means that the joints and bones do not erode or deteriorate as they do in other conditions like rheumatoid arthritis. In lupus, deformities in the hands occur for other reasons, including weakening of the tendons and ligaments, but the joints themselves are not wearing down. Arthritis is associated with joint swelling, pain, and stiffness.
6. **Heart or lung involvement**—Inflammation can occur in the lining around the heart (pericarditis) or lungs (pleuritis) and cause chest pain.
7. **Renal problems**—The word *renal* refers to the kidneys. Protein and cell casts (pieces of blood or kidney cells) in the urine can be signs that there are problems with the kidneys due to lupus.
8. **Neurological symptoms**—Lupus can affect the central nervous system (brain, spine, nerves) and cause a variety of neurological symptoms including seizures and psychosis (hallucinations, delusions, paranoia). The psychosis disappears once the lupus is stabilized, which means it was not a mental health condition but was due to lupus.
9. **Hematologic disorder**—The word *hematologic* refers to the blood. Lupus can cause blood disorders such as low red blood

cell count (anemia), low white blood cell count (leukopenia or lymphopenia), or low platelet count (thrombocytopenia).

10. **Immune system disorder**—Lab results will show the presence of antibodies against healthy cell components—anti-double-stranded DNA (anti-dsDNA); anti-Smith (anti-Sm); and antiphospholipid (aPL) antibodies that include anticardiolipin antibodies and lupus anticoagulants and can cause a false-positive syphilis test.

11. **Positive antinuclear antibody**—A positive antinuclear antibody (ANA) test is almost always present in people with lupus. Also, a positive ANA on its own does not automatically mean that someone has lupus. People with other autoimmune diseases or people with no autoimmune disease can have a positive ANA.

Others Common Symptoms

Other common lupus symptoms include:

- Debilitating fatigue is more than tiredness or exhaustion. Usually when people are tired, they sleep it off and feel refreshed the next day. Fatigue does not go away with one good night's sleep.
- Body pain, including joint and muscle pain and stiffness, may make it difficult to get out of bed or move around.
- Unexplained fevers might come and go over a period of time. They do not last a few days and then stop as with a cold or flu.
- With Raynaud's phenomenon, the fingers and toes become numb and/or turn purple or white in the cold. This can be painful.
- Forgetfulness, trouble concentrating, and trouble thinking clearly are common symptoms of lupus and are not to be confused with dementia. This is commonly referred to as lupus fog. The symptoms tend to come and go.
- Hair loss is sometimes a lupus symptom and sometimes a side effect of medication.
- A person can have lupus along with other conditions including fibromyalgia, Sjögren's syndrome, or other musculoskeletal conditions or autoimmune diseases.

Getting the Medical Care You Need

Find a Lupus Doctor

 Find a Lupus Doctor

Finding a good rheumatologist is the first step to managing lupus. Once you find one, you will meet at least once every three months. Depending on where you live, finding an experienced and conveniently located doctor could be challenging. Use the following tips to help with your search.

2 **Locate Your Local Lupus Organization**

Lupus organizations often keep lists of rheumatologists and are usually aware of their reputations. To find your local organization you can do an Internet search. Type in the name of your state and the word *lupus*.

3 Attend a Lupus Support Group, In-Person or Online

Most lupus organizations offer support groups. Support groups are invaluable for a variety of needs, including medical referrals.

4 Ask Your Primary Care Physician

Your primary care physician might know a reputable rheumatologist who has experience with lupus and can refer you. If you have other doctors, you can ask them, too.

5 Find a Member of the American College of Rheumatology

Use the American College of Rheumatology's "Find a Member" tool to locate a rheumatologist near you, both internationally and in the United States. When you contact the doctor's office, ask if they take your insurance and if they have experience with lupus.

6 Check Your Local Hospital

Check and see if your local hospital has a rheumatology department. If there is a doctor there involved in lupus research, even better. These doctors tend to be more knowledgeable and up to date.

7 Ask Your Health Insurer

Ask your health insurer for list of rheumatologists covered under your plan. Always call the doctor's office to confirm that they are in your health insurance network. Find out from your health insurer if you need a referral to see a rheumatologist.

8 Other Ways to Find a Rheumatologist Outside of the United States

Try an Internet search for a lupus organization in your country or region. You can also try finding an arthritis organization or locating a rheumatology department in a hospital near you or in a neighboring region or country. Also, search the Internet for doctors in your country or region who have done research in lupus, or who have appeared in local media discussing lupus, and contact them directly. The Lupus Foundation of America has a list of international lupus organizations and groups.

9 Narrow Down Your Search

If you are having trouble choosing from a long list, you can try narrowing down your search by the doctor's hospital affiliation, the hospital's reputation, or the presence of a lupus program. You can also narrow your search by location, gender, language spoken, and so on.

10 Chat with the Office Staff

Since there are different types of diseases that a rheumatologist can specialize in, not all rheumatologists are lupus experts. Before making your appointment, ask the office staff how many patients with lupus the doctor sees.

11 Help Educate Your Doctor about Lupus

If your only option is a doctor who does not specialize in lupus, then you need to go in prepared and informed about lupus and help educate your doctor. The Lupus Initiative has material specifically for educating health care professionals.

12 Learn about a Doctor's Research and Practice Interests

Search the Internet. A doctor's publications or a website that lists their research and practice interests might come up. See if lupus is listed.

13 Read Reviews—Learn about the Doctor's Reputation

Read online reviews to learn about a doctor's reputation, but don't place too much emphasis on some negative reviews. Are the reviews mostly positive except for a handful? Even the best doctors have people who dislike them. But if you notice the same criticism over and over, or mostly negative comments, steer clear and find someone with a better reputation.

14 Find Other Specialists

Since lupus is a systemic disease, you might need to see other types of specialists, such as a nephrologist (kidneys), cardiologist (heart), or neurologist (brain and nerves). Find other specialists the same way you would find a rheumatologist. In addition to asking a local lupus organization, you can try contacting organizations specific to that organ or disease (e.g., the National Kidney Foundation).

15 Facilitate Doctor-to-Doctor Communication

Doctor-to-doctor communication is important even for routine care, including dental exams. Some treatment options and procedures can be complicated by lupus or your medication, and your doctors need to know how to proceed based on your health status. This communication also helps prevent medication interactions.

16 | Get a Second Opinion

If your doctor is suggesting a treatment or intervention that you are unsure about, consider a second opinion. Speak with your current doctor about your concerns and discuss getting a second opinion. For an unbiased opinion, see someone at a different hospital or someone who is not affiliated with your current doctor. Find out from your insurance company if you need a referral, what its policies are about second opinions, and what it will cover.

If You are Underinsured or Uninsured

17 | Get Insured: The Health Insurance Marketplace

As of this writing, people who are uninsured or need better health care can shop for health insurance plans through their state's Health Insurance Marketplace. Speak with Marketplace representatives who can help determine what you are eligible for. They can also determine if you are eligible for Medicaid, which is free, government-funded insurance. The Marketplace can also provide contact information for a local community-based organization that can help you in applying for insurance through the Marketplace or Medicaid.

18 | Consider Your Health Care Needs

There are different levels of plans, so you should consider your health care needs, like the number of times you see a rheumatologist and other specialists each month. What are the out-of-pocket costs? You can speak with someone at your state's Marketplace to explore available options.

19 Find Out about COBRA

In many cases, immediately after you have left a place of employment, your employer will offer you COBRA, a continuation of your employer-based health insurance. The advantage of COBRA is that you can keep the plan you were on for a limited time, so you don't have to switch doctors or shop for another plan. But instead of your employer covering most of the cost, you pay the full cost of the plan, which can be high. Compare COBRA prices to Marketplace prices.

20 Other Ways to Get Insured

If you are enrolled in a college or university, find out what plans your school offers. If you are under 26, you could be added to or kept on your parents' insurance. If you are a freelancer, contact the Freelancer's Union; it offers health insurance and other benefits. Keep in mind that the Marketplace also offers health insurance for small businesses, including for sole proprietors.

21 Let Your Doctor Know if You Lost Your Insurance

If you lose your insurance or your income, let your doctor's office know. They might be able to offer sliding-scale (reduced) fees or recommendations, including where to go for cheaper lab tests or a referral to a clinic affiliated with their practice.

22 Ask Your Hospital about Charity Care

Ask your hospital about charity care. Charity care (reduced fees for medical care) is not always advertised, so asking about it is important.

23 Try a Public or Non-Profit Hospital

Try a government-funded public hospital or non-profit hospital. They have programs and benefits—including significantly reduced fees—to help people without insurance. They also may have discount pharmacies.

24 Find a Community Clinic

Many communities have low-cost or free health care centers. If this is your only option, you need to work with your doctors to make sure they know what blood tests to run, what to look for in the results, and what treatment options to prescribe since the doctor will likely be a general practitioner and not a rheumatologist.

25 Check Your Local Health Department

Typically, health departments offer services related to immunizations and sexually transmitted infections. But find out if they provide other services and programs. They could also help you find a local, free or low-cost clinic.

26 Ask Your Local Lupus Organization

Ask your local lupus organization where people without insurance can go for lupus care. They often know what to do in these situations.

27 Only Use the Emergency Room for Emergencies

Don't use the emergency room for routine lupus care. You risk not getting the right treatment or adequate follow-up care. If you do need to go to the ER, call your rheumatologist or primary health care provider immediately (or have the ER do so) so they can advise on your treatment.

Prescription Assistance

28 Ask Your Doctor

Let your doctor's office know if you don't have insurance or prescription coverage, or if you cannot afford a particular medication even with coverage. They might be able to help facilitate assistance from the pharmaceutical company. Your doctor might also be able to offer you free samples. When applicable, ask for a prescription for the generic version of the drug to help cut costs.

29 Apply for Prescription Assistance

Prescription (or patient) assistance programs will help match patients with pharmaceutical companies and organizations that offer financial assistance with the cost of a medication or with the co-payment for certain medication and treatment.

30 Call the Pharmaceutical Company

Call the pharmaceutical company directly. Many pharmaceutical companies have prescription assistance programs. Call and see if you are eligible.

31 Find Out about Emergency Grants

Check with your local lupus, arthritis, or other applicable disease organization to find out if they have emergency grants that can help if you are in a one-time bind with paying for medication or another medical bill. They might also be able to help with finding a longer-term solution.

32 Compare Prices at Pharmacies

Check with large chains like Costco, Target, and Walgreens to find out if they have prescription discount programs, sometimes called savings clubs. Compare prices between pharmacies, whether they are big chains or smaller, local stores.

33 Use a Prescription Discount Card

These are often free and can offer significant savings on prescriptions. Some have eligibility requirements. Not all cards are honored at all pharmacies. Use more than one card, if necessary, since not all cards cover all prescriptions. Compare the cost of the drug, with the discount, at a number of pharmacies.

Preparing for Your First Visit

34 Prepare for Your Visit

As you know, doctor visits are short, so it is important to make the best use of your time with any doctor you see by going in prepared. Preparation, in addition to communicating with your doctor, helps make you an active participant in your medical care. It also helps make you more aware of your medical needs, which you can then communicate with greater clarity.

35 Bring Your Medical History

Bring medical documentation, including lab and other test results. Bring a list of your other health care providers, including their contact information. List all medical conditions, treatments, and medications. Include medication doses and how often you take them. You can also bring pill bottles with you. Be sure to list any vitamins and supplements you take, because they could interact with drugs as well.

36 Don't Rely on Your Memory

Don't rely on your memory for all the questions and concerns that you want to discuss. You might forget them for many reasons, including lupus fog, anxiety, or being distracted by news you have learned during your appointment about your health status.

37 Keep a List of Questions

Keep a running list of questions in a designated place (a notebook, an app, a paper on the fridge) and write down any new lupus symptoms and/or concerns as they arise. A day or two before your appointment, organize these notes and list the most important first. Even if some of your questions go unanswered, at least you know the most important ones were addressed.

38 Find Out More about the Practice

Bring a list of questions about how the office works. How do you contact the doctor when you have a lupus flare? Will someone take the time to explain lab results, for example? If this doctor is your only option, it is still important to know these things.

39 Consider a Doctor's Bedside Manner and Other Personal Attributes

Does the doctor listen well? Seem friendly? Show genuine concern? Pay attention to your doctor's bedside manner. How important is this to you? Some people require excellent bedside manner, but others don't.

40 Acknowledge the Office Staff

The office staff is often overlooked but is a key part of your health care team. Staff members are the ones who squeeze you in for appointments when you have a lupus flare, handle your insurance, and so on. Treat them well. Find simple ways to show them gratitude. However, if they are consistently rude or difficult, let your doctor know.

Communicating with Your Doctor

41 Learn How to Communicate with Your Doctor

It takes practice for some, but it is important to learn how to communicate well with your doctor. The doctor–patient relationship is a partnership and requires two-way communication.

42 Be Assertive, Not Aggressive

Being assertive is not the same as being aggressive. It does not mean that you should yell at your doctors or treat them poorly. It means not being afraid to be open and honest in a respectful way. Don't be afraid to ask questions or follow up about lab tests or treatment or discuss questionable bedside manner, difficult office staff, or any other part of your experience.

43 Don't Worry about Being Likable

Don't worry about seeming particularly likable when you are assertive. Being particularly likable or agreeable doesn't ensure better care. Lupus is complex and requires self-advocacy through communication to ensure you are getting the best care possible.

44 Bring Someone with You to Appointments

You are absorbing a lot of information during an appointment with a doctor. When possible, take someone with you to help you communicate with your doctor, take notes, and act as general support.

45 Take Notes

If you cannot bring someone with you to help take notes, take them yourself. This will help you remember important information your doctor shared with you. Ask your doctor for help spelling the names of medication or conditions, when necessary.

46 Know Your Deal Breakers

Consider having a rule of thumb when you are trying out a new doctor. How many chances will you give a new doctor who you're unsure about? What standards do you have that your doctor has to meet? What are the deal breakers? What would lead you to look elsewhere?

47 Let Your Doctor Know if You Are Upset

If something happens between you and your doctor that upsets you, try communicating your unhappiness to your doctor before looking for someone new. Be honest with your doctor about how you feel. The response may be positive, and your relationship will move forward.

48 Use I-Statements

Use I-statements instead of you-statements. Saying, "You did this…" or "You made me feel…" is going to put the other person on the defensive and block communication. "I feel frustrated that you said that my back pain was due to my age, but this is serious and I want to look into it further. Even though I'm in my 70s, this doesn't seem normal," is an example of an I-statement. There are many examples of these online.

49 Practice with a Friend

Confronting your doctor about something that upset you can cause anxiety. It might help to talk things through with a friend or in a support group to help you figure out what to say.

50 Find Another Doctor if...

If your doctor does not respond positively to your complaint, then it might be worth your while to find a doctor you feel is a better fit. Consider the pros and cons of seeing someone else.

51 Don't Doctor Hop

Finding a doctor who will meet your needs is important, but don't doctor hop. It is really important that you find a doctor that you can see over time. Since lupus is a complex and long-term illness, consistent care is important.

52 Show Appreciation

Just as it's important for you to speak with your doctor when something is wrong, I encourage you to provide feedback when you appreciate your experiences. Good doctors are invaluable to your life with lupus, and being a doctor is not easy. A thank-you from a patient to a doctor goes a long way.

Medication and Treatment

Manage Your Medication

53 Learn about Your Medication

It's important to know what each medication is for and why it was prescribed for you. Is it a vitamin, a narcotic, an anti-inflammatory? Does it suppress your immune system? Does it protect your kidneys? Is it a painkiller? Ask your doctor to explain your medication to you.

54 Find Out about Drug Interactions

You should also speak with your doctor about possible drug interactions, known side effects, and what to do in case you experience any. Your pharmacist is also a great resource.

55 Find Out about Food Interactions

Some medications interact with certain foods or nutrients. For example, people who take the blood thinner warfarin need to be consistent with their intake of vitamin K, found in dark leafy greens and other foods. Be sure to ask your doctor or pharmacist about drug–nutrient interactions.

56 Organize Your Medication

Some people with lupus take several pills a day, sometimes dozens. Keeping track of these pills can be confusing. A pillbox can be helpful in tracking each day's worth of pills.

57 Keep Original Pill Bottles

Your original pill bottles contain instructions on how to take your medications and other important information. You may also need them when traveling. Check with your pharmacist about which medications need to be in their original containers if you take them out of the house, especially controlled substances (e.g., Xanax, codeine).

58 Keep Medication in Sight

If medication is out of sight, it is easier to forget to take. Plus, if you have lupus fog, it makes it even harder to remember. Keep your medication somewhere that you know you will see it. Pairing it with items you use every day, such as your toothbrush, could be helpful.

59 Make a Mental Note of Medication

This might be hard to do because of lupus fog, but when you take your medication, try to make a mental note, or even say aloud that you took your medication. Voicing the task helps connect you to the moment and remember it. You can even specify the day of the week and time of day. Taking pills can become so routine that we forget if we took them or not.

60 Make Note on a Calendar

Immediately after you have taken your medication, note the fact on a calendar. Keeping a calendar and pen near your pills is a great visual prompt. It reminds you to take your medication and to record the activity. And you don't have to remember where you put the calendar!

61 Use an Alarm

Use an alarm to remind you to take your medication. Cell phones and watches often have alarms that you can set to sound at the times you need to take your medication.

62 Follow Instructions

Taking a medication as instructed increases the likelihood that it will work effectively. Often, instructions related to time of day or taking with food help avoid drowsiness, insomnia, or gastrointestinal issues. Follow dosing instructions to avoid overdose and severe or life-threatening side effects. Your doctor or pharmacist can answer questions about medication instructions.

63 Don't Stop Medication without Telling Your Doctor

It is dangerous to suddenly stop certain medications, like steroids. Your doctor will instruct you on how to taper off. Speak with your doctor if you want to stop or change medication.

64 Keep a List of Medications

Keep a list of your medications folded up and stored in your wallet or purse. In addition to prescription medication, this list should include over-the-counter medication as well as vitamins and herbal or dietary supplements. Include your pharmacy's contact information. This is helpful at doctor appointments, pharmacy visits, if you have to go to urgent care or the emergency room, and simply for reference and keeping track of your medications. Update the list when necessary.

65 Consider Medical Identification Jewelry

Use a medical identification bracelet, necklace, or wallet card that contains such key information as "Lupus," "On Multiple Medications," or "Allergic to Sulfa Drugs," for example. Some jewelry IDs include the phone number of the company that issues them, so that emergency responders can call and obtain important medical information.

66 See an Eye Doctor if Taking Hydroxychloroquine (Plaquenil)

Hydroxychloroquine is one of the safest and most common drugs used to treat lupus. It does, however, come with the rare possibility of retina toxicity, and people who take it need to have their eyes checked every six months. Before taking the drug they need to get a baseline of their vision, which will be used for comparison in later examinations. Speak with your rheumatologist for more information.

67 What to Do if You Are Having Side Effects

If you are having side effects, it is important to call your doctor's office, let them know, and request to speak with the doctor as soon as possible. Your doctor should instruct you on what to do next. If you cannot reach your doctor, call your pharmacist and speak with your doctor later. If you need to stop taking the medication, you need to be instructed on how to do so safely. If you are having severe side effects, you can go to urgent care or, if very severe, call 911 immediately.

68 Could Unusual Symptoms Be Medication Side Effects?

If you are having symptoms that are not caused by lupus or another medical condition, then medication side effects or drug interactions may be the culprit. Speak with your doctor and pharmacist about this possibility.

69 Afraid of Possible Side Effects?

Those wary about taking medication should speak with their doctor about the risks and benefits of taking or not taking a certain medication. Often, the risk is that your lupus can get worse or dangerous, and it is best to take the medication. If there is a certain medication that worries you, find out if your doctor can prescribe something else.

70 Beware of Internet Reviews about Medication

If you look up other people's experiences with medication, I guarantee that you will find endless horror stories. It is not an accurate representation of the general experience with a medication. Try not to let Internet reviews be the basis of your decision.

71 Try Out a Medication for Yourself

You have already spoken with your doctor and pharmacist about the risks and benefits. Every person has an individual response to medication, and if you feel that the benefits outweigh the risks, the only way to know how a medication will work with your body is to try it for yourself.

Complementary and Alternative Treatment

72 Consider Complementary Treatment

Complementary treatments are additions to your routine medical (allopathic) care, as opposed to alternative treatments that replace medical care. Complementary treatments can help improve your quality of life, health, and overall well-being. These often include therapies that use the mind or body to feel better physically and mentally.

73 Find the Right Complementary Treatment for You

Examples of complementary treatments are massage therapy, physical or occupational therapy, restorative yoga, water aerobics and water tai chi, tai chi, qigong, meditation, creative visualization, aromatherapy, and acupuncture. Different therapies are associated with benefits that include pain relief, less stiffness, and stress reduction. Always discuss these with your doctor before starting one.

74 Modify Exercises

If you are taking a class such as yoga, let the instructor know that you need help modifying some of the poses or movements. Stop if you are in pain and let your instructor, therapist, or practitioner know.

75 When to Avoid Massage Therapy

It's important not to get a massage while you are in the middle of a flare or if you have a rash. Deep tissue massage can worsen lupus symptoms. It's important to let your massage therapist know what medical conditions you have and if you are experiencing any symptoms.

76 Find a Responsible Practitioner

If you are going to see a complementary treatment practitioner, find out if they have experience with lupus. Find out the severity of the lupus they've seen, and the challenges and successes they've had in treating others with lupus. Always let them know what medication you take, your current symptoms, and any other relevant health information.

77 Don't Take Risks with Alternative Treatment

Medication that your doctor prescribes has undergone rigorous research and testing. This is not the case with alternative treatments. Some have been studied and found to be ineffective or dangerous; others have not been studied, which makes them risky. Once an alternative treatment is researched, tested, and found to be effective and safe, it is approved for use and no longer considered alternative.

78 Tell Your Doctor about Wanting to Stop Medication

If you are having a negative experience with your medication and want to replace it with an alternative treatment, speak with your doctor about these experiences and concerns. Don't start an alternative treatment and stop medication without your doctor's knowledge. Work with your doctor to find a solution. Stopping medication can be dangerous for people with lupus. Lupus medication has saved many lives.

79 Don't Assume There's a Secret Cure

If lupus could be cured by a supplement or special diet, you would know. Finding the cure is a research scientist's dream. Don't believe claims that there is a secret or simple cure. Often, people making these claims have an agenda, like selling you a product or service that hasn't been tested for safety or effectiveness.

80 Don't Take Someone's Word for It

If someone tells you that you should stop taking your medication and try an alternative treatment such as a special diet or supplement, don't take their word for it, no matter how much they say it has done for them. You don't know their situation, health status, or the whole story. For every person that claims they cured lupus with an alternative treatment, there are many more who experienced no results or got sicker, sometimes dangerously so.

81 Do Your Research

If you are curious about the uses, effectiveness, and safety of an herb, vitamin, or other dietary supplement or alternative or complementary treatment, look it up on the National Institutes of Health's National Center for Complementary and Integrative Health website. It provides summaries based on research.

82 Continue to See Your Doctor

Given the serious risks of not taking medication, if you refuse medication, I strongly urge you to continue to see a rheumatologist at least every three months. This way, you can continue monitoring your health status and lupus activity levels with lab tests. Without this monitoring, lupus activity could increase quietly and might not manifest until significant damage is done. The goal is prevention and intervention as early as possible.

83 When It's Okay to Add an Alternative Treatment

Sometimes, if a doctor thinks a particular alternative treatment is safe and has heard enough positive feedback about it from patients, they might agree that it is okay for you to try. But this does not mean you should stop more conventional medications.

84 Speak with Your Doctor about Treatment Additions

Always speak with your doctor before making changes or additions to your treatment, such as herbs, vitamins, and other dietary supplements. Sometimes they can interact with medication.

85 If You Are Going to Work with an Herbalist...

If you are going to work with an herbalist, find a responsible, reputable practitioner who has experience with lupus and uses pure ingredients from reputable sources. Ideally, your herbalist and rheumatologist should communicate with each other, or you should work closely with your doctor about your herbalist's plan. An herbalist does not replace a rheumatologist.

86 Know the Purity of Vitamins and Supplements

In the United States, the Federal Drug Administration does not monitor the purity of herbs, vitamins, and other dietary supplements. Sometimes there are toxins like lead in herbs, or supplements are fakes (labeling fraud). This can be both dangerous and a waste of money. Speak with your doctor or pharmacist about which brands to use.

87 Don't Assume Herbs, Vitamins, and Supplements Are Chemical Free

There is a misconception that if something comes from nature, it is chemical free. Herbs, vitamins, and supplements contain natural and/or human-made chemicals. Not all chemicals are bad. Natural is not always good. Often, it's the dose that matters. For example, salt is a naturally occurring chemical that we use all the time with food but, in large doses, is toxic to the human body. Of course, some chemicals, natural or human made, are toxic at any dose.

88 Don't Take Alfalfa, Sulfa-Containing Drugs, or Echinacea

Alfalfa, sulfa-containing drugs (e.g., some antibiotics), and echinacea may increase lupus activity. Echinacea can also interact with certain lupus medications. Speak with your doctor for more information.

89 Talk with Your Doctor about Approved Supplements

Some vitamins and supplements are commonly taken by people with lupus, including vitamin D and calcium (bone health), B vitamins (energy levels), and omega-3 fatty acids (may help reduce inflammation). Speak with your doctor about approved supplements, possible drug interactions, and how much to take. Also, if your doctor is able to prescribe vitamins or supplements for you, your health insurance may cover the cost.

90 Ask about Calcium

Steroids can cause bone loss, so it is important to ask your doctor if you need a bone-density exam, and if you need to take a calcium supplement. Among other things, calcium is important for bone health.

91 Get Your Vitamin D Levels Checked

Ask your doctor to check your vitamin D levels. Vitamin D is needed to help your body absorb calcium, so they are often taken together. But also, as of this writing, there have been studies showing a possible relationship between low vitamin D levels and increased lupus activity. Speak with your doctor about the research.

Real versus Fake Science

92 Learn How to Tell Real Science from Fake (Pseudo) Science

There is a lot of false information in the world, especially on the Internet, which is a problem when you are trying to understand lupus and lupus treatment. It is important to develop the skills to figure out what is real science and what is fake (pseudo) science.

93 Is It a Trustworthy Website?

Just because the name of a website sounds legitimate doesn't mean that it is. Anyone can say anything and claim that it's true, including on the Internet. Ask yourself where they get their information. Do they back up their claims with reliable sources? Also, search the Internet to learn more about a questionable website. If it's controversial or spreads inaccurate information, you'll find out.

94 Beware of Fake News or Joke Websites

Some websites purposely put out fake news as a joke and do not make any claims that what they publish is true. Sometimes, however, readers are unaware of this and mistake satire for real news. Examples of this include *The Onion*, the *Daily Currant*, and *World News Daily Report*.

95 Don't Rely on the Popular Media

Don't rely on the popular media, including daily news outlets and popular magazines, to accurately summarize research findings. They often skew or exaggerate the information to support a certain angle or agenda.

96 Go to the Source

If a research article is available for free online, consider trying to read it. Try to understand how the study was implemented, its strengths and weaknesses, and the final conclusions. If the numbers and jargon are confusing, read the introduction and the discussion. They are often written in plainer language and contain useful information.

97 Find Reliable Summaries of the Original Source

Reading a research paper is challenging for many people. Find a legitimate science- or medicine-based source that summarizes the research article, like *Lupus News Today* and *MedPage Today*. You can also call a lupus organization or bring an article to your doctor for help understanding the research and findings.

98 Seek Out Other Reliable Sources

The National Institutes of Health websites rely on solid research evidence. Reputable disease organizations have their material reviewed by trusted medical professionals, academic journals, and research institutes. Information coming out of distinguished universities often comes from professors who are experts in their fields. Well-known hospitals are excellent sources of information. If they have a program for lupus, even better.

99 Don't Assume an MD or PhD Is a Reliable Source

If anyone with an advanced degree—such as an MD or PhD—makes controversial claims or statements that sound too good to be true, question their trustworthiness. This includes doctors who claim lupus can be cured by taking their supplements or by following dietary advice in one of their books. They are trying to sell a product. Quackwatch.org is a site that can help you figure out if someone is untrustworthy.

100 Who's the Author? And What Is Their Agenda?

Having a political or business agenda can skew how information is presented. Do research on authors, including doctors. What evidence is there to support your trust in them or in their claims? Usually, being affiliated with a reputable institution is a good sign.

101 Check the Date

How old is the information? Make sure it's current. Benlysta—the first drug approved for lupus in over 50 years—was approved by the FDA in 2011. Articles on lupus treatment written before 2011 likely would not include information on this important development. An online search of the topic using the current year (or past few years) can help you find the most recent information.

102 Find Out if It Is a Hoax or False Claim

Search online with the title or topic of a story to see if it comes up as a hoax. When you search for an article online, do any other reliable sources come up? If it is breaking news, then local news outlets would share the same information. Does the story sound wild, unusual, or too good to be true? Hint: be suspicious of anything that claims to be the cure for lupus.

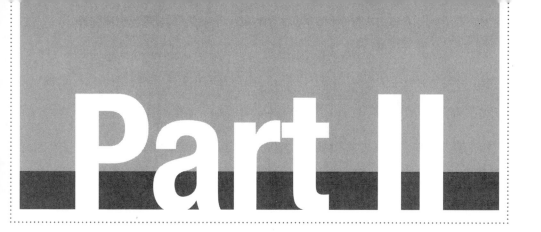

Living Well

You Are Not Alone

Find Support

103 Find Support

For many, support is critical to living well with lupus. Support can be useful in reducing a sense of isolation, helping you feel understood, providing a sense of belonging, and providing mentorship on how to best cope with lupus. In addition to emotional support, groups are a great source of information about lupus, local doctors, and other resources.

104 Speak with a Friend

You might already know someone with lupus or another chronic illness. Some chronic illnesses share similar symptoms such as pain and fatigue. It can be very helpful to have a friend to speak with who understands what it's like to live with a chronic illness.

105 Find a Support Group

The best way to find an in-person support group is through your local lupus organization. You can also do an Internet search for telephone or online support groups, or join one on social media, like Facebook.

106 Your First Support Group

If possible, speak to the group facilitator before you attend. Ask questions:. How big is the group? How often and where does it meet? How long are the meetings? What are the group rules? Do I have to share or can I just listen? What do people usually talk about? Is it okay to bring a friend or family member?

107 Expect a Variety of Personalities

Different people have different personalities, and having lupus in common won't change that. You will identify with some and not so much with others. A good facilitator will do his or her best to manage different personalities and keep the group supportive and respectful.

108 Expect to Hear Differences in Lupus

No two people with lupus have the same exact symptoms. Severity of its symptoms can vary widely. Do not assume that the way lupus manifests in someone else will be what you should expect for yourself.

109 Meet with a Psychotherapist

If you want more frequent or individualized support, or if you want to talk more deeply about feelings and experiences, seeing a psychotherapist might be a good option. People typically meet with therapists once a week if it is covered by their health insurance.

110 Find a Psychotherapist

You can find a therapist through your health insurance company or at your local community clinic or hospital. Your lupus organization, doctors, or support group members may also have good recommendations.

111 Choosing a Therapist

When considering therapists, ask how much experience they have with lupus or chronic illness. Be sure they are licensed mental health practitioners (i.e., social workers, marriage and family therapists, psychologists, or psychiatrists). Find out if they are talk therapists who focus more on the emotional experience, or cognitive behavioral therapists who focus more on reframing the thoughts and behaviors that make coping a challenge. Find out if they provide video chats or phone sessions for days you need to stay home. Just like searching for doctors, it might take a few tries before you find the right fit.

Lupus and Grief

112 Grieving Is Okay and Natural

Grief is how people respond to loss, whether the loss is death related or not. There are many losses associated with lupus. It is okay and natural to be sad and angry about these losses, to miss them, and to grieve them.

113 Grieve When You Need to Grieve

People with lupus grieve when they first learn they have lupus and are adjusting to the losses, when they experience changes in their health status, or at other times in their lives. Grieve when you need to grieve.

114 Seek Professional Support for Grief

Speaking with a professional to help you through the grief process can be invaluable. You can speak with a psychotherapist who specializes in grief or with a grief counselor. When screening therapists and counselors, ask about their experience with loss and grief related to chronic illness.

Lupus and Depression

115 Grief or Depression? Know That They Are Different

While grief is an expected reaction to loss that usually eases over time, depression is a chronic mental health condition. Sometimes their symptoms, such as intense sadness, look very similar. People with depression can also grieve, and people who grieve can also be depressed, but they are not the same. If you are not sure which you are experiencing, speaking with a therapist can be helpful in sorting this out.

116 Lupus and Depression, Seek Support

A person with lupus could have had depression before the lupus diagnosis. Understandably, a person might also become depressed because of the challenges of living with lupus. If you feel depressed, seek support from a psychotherapist. Without treatment, both lupus and depression can become dangerous. With treatment and support, both conditions can be managed.

117 Depression or Lupus? Speak with Your Rheumatologist

If you are feeling depressed, it's important to tell your rheumatologist so you can work together to figure out the cause. Depression can also be related to the physical impact of lupus on your body or a medication side effect.

118 What to Do in an Emotional Crisis

If you are in an emotional crisis where you feel overwhelmed, that life is not worth living, or are having thoughts of self-harm or suicide, please tell someone. You should reach out right away to a friend or family member, your therapist, or any of your doctors. You can also reach out to a crisis hotline. They are open 24/7/365. Call 1-800-273-8255 or text the word ANSWER to 839863. These types of feelings don't tend to happen just once, so hopefully you will ultimately connect with a good therapist who you will meet with regularly, and in that time create a safety plan together.

119 If You Are in Immediate Danger

If you feel you are in immediate danger of hurting yourself, do not act on your thoughts. Call 911 on your own or call the crisis hotline and ask them to call for you. If you can find someone you trust, ask them to stay with you until you are admitted into the hospital.

120 If You Are Worried about the Hospital

If you are worried about going to a hospital for feeling suicidal, know that it is a temporary place to stay until you are safe. Keeping you alive and safe is the main priority, just as if it were a physical health emergency.

Men with Lupus

121 Getting a Diagnosis

No matter what anyone tells you, men get lupus, too. If a doctor has said that you can't have lupus because you are a man, find a new rheumatologist with lupus experience, or bring educational material to your current doctor if that is your only option.

122 Know That You Are Not a Man with a Woman's Disease

You are a person with lupus of any gender. While it is true that most people with lupus are women, anyone can get lupus, including men.

123 Find Support

Because some men with a lupus diagnosis feel alienated, it is important to find support. A good group will welcome you regardless of your gender. Many lupus-related experiences are universal, and you have more in common than not. You might meet other men with lupus, too. Seeing a therapist is a more private option.

124 Talk about Your Experience as a Man

Consider sharing your feelings about being a man with lupus, even if that's difficult to do. You could, for example, talk about how the lupus community sometimes forgets about men and how that frustrates you. For some men, gender identity is tied to being physically strong, providing for their families, and being hard workers. Lupus may impact your ability to do these things, possibly affecting your sense of self-worth.

125 Express Your Emotions

For a variety of personal and/or cultural reasons, some men feel uncomfortable expressing their emotions. Realize that expressing yourself is a part of managing and coping with your illness. Also realize that you are human and have a wide range of emotions that may be heightened or stirred by this disease. Your feelings are valid. Coping with lupus is complicated and challenging regardless of gender.

126 Seek Out Other Men with Lupus

Some men find comfort and feel less alienated when connected with other men with lupus. Your local lupus organization or rheumatologist might know other men with lupus whom they could connect you to (with the other person's permission, of course). You could also find other men with lupus, autoimmune disease, or chronic illness online in support groups or on message boards.

Maintaining a Healthy Lifestyle

Lupus and Nutrition

127 There Is No Lupus Diet

There is no specific diet for people with lupus. Eating a nutritious diet, though, can only help your body, which is already taxed by the experience of autoimmune disease. Some people find that certain foods cause flares and avoid eating them. Diet, however, will not cure lupus.

128 Know Your Health Risks

People with lupus are at an increased risk for heart disease and stroke, and steroids increase the chance of weight gain and diabetes. Speak with your doctor about dietary recommendations associated with these risks. For example, people with kidney involvement should watch their salt intake.

129 Eat Real Food

Real foods include fruits, vegetables, whole grains, nuts, seeds, beans, lean meats, dairy, and fish. When possible, and within your budget, eat organic. Some foods, such as apples and potatoes, can be peeled to help avoid pesticides even if they aren't organic.

130 Stay Away from Processed Foods

Processed foods include foods that are far from their natural state, stripped of their nutrients, and loaded with additives. Examples of processed foods are candy, potato chips, white rice, white bread, white sugar, fast food, imitation meats, cold cuts, artificial sweeteners, low-fat processed foods, juice beverages (not 100% juice), and soda. The more you avoid processed foods and replace them with real, natural foods, the better.

131 Just Do Your Best with Diet

Sometimes eating a nutritious diet can be challenging when you have to deal with fatigue and financial constraints. Do the best you can without negatively judging yourself. If your insurance covers it, seeing a nutritionist for guidance can be helpful.

132 Listen to Your Body

There is not enough research to say which foods are bad for lupus and which are good. Listen to your body and how it reacts to certain foods. For example, popular lore says that nightshades such as eggplant exacerbate lupus symptoms. Yet there is no research to support this claim, and some people with lupus eat nightshades with no side effects.

133 Address Food Allergies and Food Sensitivity

An allergist can test you for food allergies. Allergies are specific, immune-system responses to food and can sometimes be life threatening. Food sensitivity is an unpleasant bodily response that is less severe than an allergic reaction. Some people without allergies find that certain foods trigger an increase in lupus symptoms. If you don't have food allergies and suspect that food is a major trigger, speak with your doctor and, if possible, a nutritionist. You may want to explore the option of an elimination diet.

134 Figure Out if the Elimination Diet Is Right for You

Elimination diets are temporary, generally safe, and possibly useful in pinpointing those foods your body cannot tolerate. It is important, however, to maintain proper nutrition during the diet since you will be cutting out food groups. This diet can be challenging and restrictive, and is not recommended for people with a history of eating disorders or food phobia. It should be done under the supervision of a doctor.

135 Keep a Food Journal

Elimination diet or not, if you notice that you don't feel well after eating certain foods, make note of this in your journal. Include the foods you ate and the symptoms you experienced. If you notice a pattern over time, tell your doctor. There are many food diaries, journaling apps, and worksheets available for free on the Internet that can help you to keep track.

Strive for a Healthy Lifestyle

136 Don't Smoke

Smoking can increase disease severity and activity, and decrease treatment effectiveness. It can also increase the risk of multiple cardiovascular issues, respiratory infection, and organ damage. Secondhand smoke should also be avoided. If you need help quitting, there are many resources online, including hotlines and programs that provide free nicotine patches.

137 Don't Drink Alcohol in Excess

Speak with your doctor or pharmacist about alcohol and medication interactions. In addition to commonly known cardiovascular and liver problems associated with drinking in excess, alcohol can decrease bone health and increase the risk of digestive problems, especially if you take NSAIDs. Some people report an increase in lupus symptoms when drinking alcohol. If you experience this, document it in your food journal and tell your doctor.

138 Exercise When Possible

Many forms of low-impact exercise—such as walking, swimming, and low-impact aerobics—are great complementary treatments, but working out can be hard when you are fatigued or in pain. Take advantage of the times when you feel good to exercise. Exercise can help decrease pain and stiffness, improve muscle strength, and reduce stress, and in turn this can lead to feeling well enough to exercise more often.

139 Other Tips for Exercising

Check with your doctor about the best exercise plan for you and how to prevent injury. Don't do too much too fast; you want to avoid increased fatigue or joint pain. Listen to your body, especially if it is telling you to stop, slow down, or try something different. Build up your stamina gradually. Wear sunscreen if you exercise outdoors. Always stay hydrated.

140 Try to Get Enough Sleep

If you have trouble sleeping, speak with your doctor about sleep apnea, bedtime behavior changes, or medicinal sleep aids. Does poor sleep cause pain and fatigue or does pain and fatigue cause poor sleep? The answer is unclear. What is clear, however, is that sleep is important for managing mood, thinking and memory, and lupus symptoms.

141 Track Your Sleep

Keep a sleep diary to track your sleeping patterns. This might help you figure out what is contributing to poor sleep. There are many sleep diary resources, including online apps.

Managing Stress

Plan Ahead for a Flare

142 Plan Ahead for a Flare

To reduce stress and other problems during a flare, it helps to plan ahead. Think about what happens to your life when you have a flare. Where will you need assistance? How can you set things up in advance of a flare so you don't find yourself in a jam?

143 Revisit the List of Your Medical Information

Revisit that list you took to your doctor that includes information about your medications, health conditions, doctors you see, and medication allergies. This list is helpful in the event of a severe flare that leads you to the ER.

144 Make Your Medical Information Easy to Find

Carry a smaller version of this list in your wallet and keep a copy in a place that would be visible to emergency responders— taped to the back of the front door, for instance. Put the paperwork in an envelope and label it in large letters (e.g., <u>For EMS</u>). Medical identification jewelry would be helpful, too.

145 Make a List of Your Bills

If you are in the hospital or stuck in bed, your bills are probably the last thing on your mind. Make a list of all the bills you have to pay and their due dates. Keeping a folder with a paper copy of each bill is helpful, too. If you are in a flare, the last thing you want to do is rely on your memory to remember which bills to pay.

146 Use Auto-Pay

If you pay bills online, auto-payments are an option. For each bill, enter a monthly payment date, and your money will be automatically transferred from your bank. Be sure that you have enough money in your account to cover the payments.

147 Make a List of Household Needs

Think about your daily necessities—things you must have, activities you must do—and make a list. You'll need food to eat. If you have young kids, they need to be bathed, dressed, fed, taken to school, and picked up. If you have pets, dogs need to be walked, and cats need to have the litter changed, and so on.

148 Ask for Help

Ask for help from people who seem supportive, including family, friends, and neighbors. People often want to help but don't know how. Helping you when you are in a flare gives them concrete ways to be supportive. It is also a way to open up communication about your experience with lupus.

149 Commitments Outside of the Home

Make a list of your commitments outside of the home, such as where you work, volunteer, or regularly attend appointments or other activities. Again, include all necessary contact information. This is helpful if you have to let someone know you will be absent because of a flare.

150 Don't Insist on a Perfect Plan

Not everyone has the same resources and support system, so you might not have a solution for every need. Do the best you can. No plan is perfect. Anything you prepare for in advance is helpful. Support groups are also great places to seek suggestions for meeting these needs.

151 Self-Care during a Flare

Reducing stress by preparing to cover your commitments during a flare is a great self-care tool, but don't neglect your own personal comfort. Who can you talk with on the phone for support or a good laugh? Who can pay you a visit if you can't go out? What can you do so you don't get bored? How can you pamper yourself? How can others pamper you? With lupus, pampering yourself is a prescription for self-care, not a luxury.

152 Put It All Together

Put together all your lists and documents—your medical information, your bills and their due dates, contact information for commitments outside of the home, and strategies for addressing responsibilities in the home. If friends, family, or neighbors have agreed to help you, this should be indicated. Include any other information you feel is important.

153 Keep Everything in One Place

Keep a copy of these documents in one safe place. Make sure you will be able to find it or let someone else know where it is. You can also keep a password-protected version on your computer.

154 Keep Your Support System Involved

Sharing and reviewing all or some of these documents with one or two trusted and supportive loved ones will help keep them involved and aware of your life with lupus. But it's best to keep sensitive medical and financial information private.

Manage Energy Levels

155 Learn Your Energy Limits

Because of fatigue, you have a limited amount of energy. Be strategic about how you use it. Listen to your body when it tells you that your energy is running low, and that you need a rest. Overdoing it can increase fatigue or other lupus symptoms.

156 Pace Yourself

How exhilarating it is when you have felt tired for days and suddenly feel energized! The temptation is to squeeze in as much as possible before fatigue sets in again. Do your best to pace yourself to prevent an increase in symptoms. Some people focus on the most important thing on their to-do list. Others decide to do something fun.

157 Learn How to Say, "No"

Learn to say, "No"—to both yourself and others—when you sense that pushing yourself will cause fatigue the next day. This can be very hard to do and will take practice, but doing too much will do no good for your health.

158 Get to Know Your Best Time of Day

Some people are early birds; others need to sleep in. Figure out if there is a time of day when you have peak energy and function best. Take this into consideration for daily tasks and chores and when making plans.

159 Try to Plan Your Days

Try to plan your days so that you don't pack too much in. Once you understand your energy limits, you will get a better sense of how much you can handle on an average, flare-free day.

160 Learn to Rest

If you have overdone it, you need to rest. If you feel like there are so many things you want to do, but just can't get up and do them, you need to rest. You're not being lazy. You are managing your health. Get the rest you need. Think of it like a prescription—one you shouldn't miss. Scheduling a daily time to rest helps, too.

161 Practice Time-Management Skills

Learn how to make the most of your time when you have the energy to be active. The Internet has plenty of information on time management. For example, don't multitask, and learn how to prioritize your to-do list.

162 Be Forgiving of Yourself

You will run out of energy and not be able to do everything you want to do. You will overextend yourself and end up fatigued the next day. Don't punish yourself for this. Forgive yourself, move forward, and try a different approach next time. Managing lupus is a lot of work, and no one handles it perfectly.

More Stress Management Tools

163 Manage Your Stress Levels

Stress is linked to health problems for everyone. But it's important for people with lupus to manage their stress levels because stress can trigger a flare. Planning ahead for a flare and implementing energy and other stress management tools will help you manage your stress levels.

164 Practice Gratitude

It can be easy to dwell on the ways lupus has harshly impacted your life. One way to manage these thoughts is to make a conscious effort to focus on what is going right. There are many ways to practice gratitude, such as gratitude journaling, keeping a gratitude jar, or sending thank-you cards to people you appreciate. There are also helpful websites and apps about practicing gratitude.

165 Find Comfort in Spirituality and Religion

Not everyone is spiritual, and that's okay: There are many ways to cope. Many people with lupus who are spiritual, however, believe that their spirituality plays a big role in coping. It often helps to feel supported and guided by a higher power.

166 Meditate

Meditation helps improve memory and concentration and reduce stress. It can also help diminish one's perception of pain. There are many different types of meditation. Try out different ones. You can find free videos online.

167 Practice Mindfulness

Mindfulness helps us live in the present. People can experience a lot of anxiety from the unpredictability of lupus—not knowing how they will feel day to day, how the disease will progress, when a flare will happen. Focusing on the present helps prevent your mind from becoming overwhelmed with worries of the future.

168 Do Things You Find Enjoyable

Seems obvious, doesn't it? Yet, some lupus patients have trouble allowing themselves a break from their responsibilities. Engaging in an enjoyable activity, even if it is simple, can bring meaning to your day, improve your mood, and keep you focused on something positive and pleasing.

169 Be Creative

Participating in the arts can be therapeutic in many wonderful ways. It keeps your mind engaged and open to new ways of seeing the world. The process of creating something new and original can be exciting—and the product itself a source of pride and achievement. So pick up a camera, write a blog, join a local theater group or vocal ensemble— whatever inspires you— and enjoy all the benefits of being creative.

170 Connect with Nature

Connecting with nature can help clear your mind and reduce tension. Even if you live in an urban environment, you can find a few elements of nature to closely observe—like the feel of a tree, its grooves and patterns, or the types of birds that are perched in the trees. Listen to the relaxing sounds of nature such as the rhythm and roll of ocean waves. You can find free videos of this online.

171 Explore Your Passions

Spend time doing what you love. It can be hard when lupus has affected your ability to do certain activities. Explore other hobbies and interests. Have you wanted to learn more about a certain subject or skill set? Consider taking a course at your local library, community center, or YMCA, and if you take a little time searching you can find free online courses offered by many top universities. You never know what new joys you will discover!

172 Laugh

Laugh as much as possible! Laughing provides an emotional buffer between you and the challenges of living with lupus. Plus, laughter is known to reduce tension and pain, and boost endorphins—the happiness hormones.

173 Volunteer

Volunteering helps you to understand that your entire life isn't about lupus. You can still be helpful and productive. You can learn new skills and knowledge and feel good about helping others. It also takes your mind off lupus and lets you feel less isolated as you build positive relationships with others.

Managing Lupus Fog

174 Write It Down

The number one tool for managing lupus fog is to write down as much as possible, and as soon as possible. Don't assume you will remember something.

175 Keep a Notepad

Keep a small notepad with you at all times so that you have one central place to write things down, or use the notes section on your phone.

176 Keep a Calendar

Schedule your daily tasks on a calendar, including doctor appointments. Schedule reminders in advance of appointments and tasks as well, and include any important information, like time and location of the appointment, people's names and numbers, and the nature of the appointment. This way, you won't have to go looking for this information later.

177 Sticky Notes

Use sticky notes strategically. If there is something you need to remember, put a sticky note where you will likely see it as a reminder, such as the bathroom mirror or front door.

178 Use Alarms

Use alarms to help you remember tasks, appointments, and taking medication. Most cell phones have built-in alarms that you can set. Some watches have alarms, as well.

179 Leave Yourself a Voicemail

If you happen to find yourself without a notepad, call yourself and leave a voicemail reminder about whatever it is you don't want to forget. Or send yourself a text or e-mail.

180 Take Pictures

Use your camera or cell-phone camera to take photos of anything you want to remember. You can use the photo instead of a written reminder. Take a photo of a support-group flyer hanging on a wall, for example. Taking screenshots of information from your phone or Internet browser, such as an address you looked up, is helpful too.

181 Declutter

Taking pictures helps reduce the amount of paper you carry, which helps you declutter. Try to get rid of any unnecessary paper or items that you don't use or really want. You will have less to keep track of in your home and will be more organized.

182 Stay Organized

It's hard to stay organized while dealing with fatigue and lupus fog. When possible, organize one thing at a time. For example, label your files one day. File your documents on another.

183 Be Consistent

Keep your belongings in the same, obvious places all the time. For example, keep your keys in a basket by the front door and always put them there when you get home.

184 Make To-Do Lists

Keep track of your important daily tasks with to-do lists. Be sure that you take your notepad with you at bedtime since we tend to remember important things to add to our to-do lists while in bed. You don't want to drag yourself out of bed to look for paper and a pen.

185 Breathe

When you find yourself getting frustrated by lupus fog, pause and take some deep breaths. This will help relax both your mind and body.

186 Find Humor in the Situation

Did lupus fog cause you to do something totally ridiculous? Being able to laugh at yourself is a great way to cope. Share the story with your support group. Others will relate.

187 Remember, It's Not Your Fault

Lupus fog is not your fault. There is nothing wrong with you as a person because you can't think clearly sometimes, or because you are more forgetful. Lupus fog is not a sign of diminished intelligence, either. Lupus fog is caused by lupus. Be gentle with yourself. You are doing the best you can.

188 Keep a Log

Keep a log of when you experience lupus fog. Include as many details as possible, including the date and what occurred. Notice whether symptoms worsen or stay the same over time. Include strategies that help you with these symptoms. Share this log with your doctor.

189 Talk with Your Doctor

Always tell your rheumatologist if you are experiencing symptoms of lupus fog. If you notice that you are having an increase in symptoms or their intensity, let your rheumatologist know. They might refer you to a neurologist or neuropsychologist familiar with lupus for further testing.

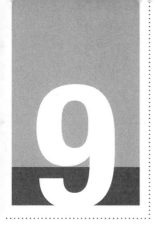

Lupus on the Outside

190 Feeling Self-Conscious Is Normal

Although there are many internal manifestations of lupus, it is often the external signs of the disease that are most difficult to cope with. It is normal to feel self-conscious about the way lupus impacts your personal appearance. Allow yourself to process these feelings and share them with your support system.

191 Don't Take Over-the-Counter Hair Loss Medication

These treatments are not for your condition. Talk with your rheumatologist to try to determine the cause of the hair loss and how to treat it. The hair loss may be due to a flare, a medication side effect, or something unrelated, such as a vitamin deficiency or hormone imbalance.

192 Ask if the Hair Loss Is Permanent

Some people worry that hair loss is permanent. Sometimes it is. Sometimes it is not, depending on the cause and whether there is scarring. Ask your doctor whether they think your hair will grow back.

193 Talk with Your Doctor about Biotin

Some claim that biotin (vitamin B7) will help with hair growth, including for people with lupus. However, there is not enough evidence to back this up. A biotin deficiency is rare and can result in hair thinning, but this is not lupus related. If biotin is something you're considering, speak with your rheumatologist first about safety, drug interactions, effectiveness, and dose before actually trying it.

194 Consider Hair Accessories

The least expensive way to handle hair loss is to use a hair accessory such as a wrap, scarf, or hat. The Internet is full of online stores that specialize in wraps and scarves for hair loss, as well as tutorials on how to use them.

195 Try a New Hairdo

A hairstylist could help by styling or cutting your hair in such a way that hides hair loss or makes hair look fuller. A new hairdo can go a long way.

196 Find Out if Hair Extensions or a Weave is Right for You

It's best to work with a hairstylist who has experience with hair loss because, depending on the method, weaves or extensions could increase hair loss. If you are a good candidate and have the right hairstylist, however, these are good options. But keep in mind that extensions require upkeep and maintenance. Check with your hairstylist to get an esitimated monthly cost.

197 Try a Wig

This could be an expensive option, depending on the quality of the wig. A good wig can, however, look remarkably authentic and natural.

198 Surgery

If you have lost a lot of hair permanently, and the other options are not to your liking, you could speak with your rheumatologist about surgical options like hair transplantation. Be sure to educate yourself fully on all aspects of this procedure.

199 Try Camouflage Makeup

Try makeup to cover scarring, discoloration, or other lupus-related skin changes. There are brands, like Dermablend®, that offer makeup specifically for this purpose. It is referred to as camouflage makeup.

200 Ask for a Free Sample

Before spending a lot of money on cosmetics, find out if you can get a free sample or makeup consultation to make sure that a certain brand works well with your skin. Let the clerk or consultant know if you tend to be makeup sensitive, so they can suggest the best option for you.

201 Anyone Can Try These

Some people might think that these hair and makeup suggestions are for women only, They are not. Anyone can benefit from these tips.

202 Wear Sunscreen

What should you look for in a sunscreen? Three things: broad-spectrum protection against both UVA and UVB rays, an SPF of at least 30, and water resistance.

203 Don't Forget to Protect Your Lips

Many people forget that their lips are exposed to the sun and neglect to protect them. Remember to use lip balm daily, with an SPF of at least 15.

204 Apply Sunscreen Correctly

Remember to put sunscreen on about 15 to 20 minutes before you go outside so it has time to absorb into your skin. Reapply every couple of hours or after swimming or sweating a lot. And make sure to use enough to thoroughly cover all exposed skin.

205 Wear Makeup with UVA and UVB Protection

If you wear makeup, it's best to use products with UVA and UVB protection. If your makeup doesn't have sun protection, you should wear both sunscreen and makeup.

206 Other Ways to Protect Yourself from the Sun

Sun-blocking clothing with UV protection, wide-brimmed hats, long sleeves, umbrellas, and walking in the shade help shield you from the sun. Also, when you get a new prescription, ask your doctor or pharmacist if the medication increases sun sensitivity.

207 Talk with Your Doctor about Weight Fluctuation

If you are gaining weight or losing weight, let your rheumatologist know. They can help determine if it's a medication side effect, lupus related, or something else.

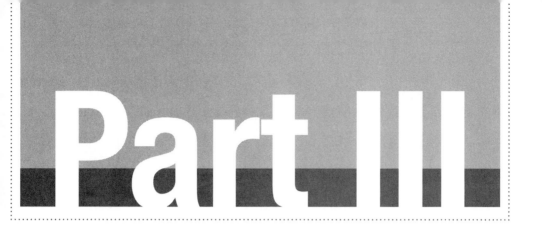

Lupus and Personal
Relationships

Family and Friends

Support from Friends and Family

208 Ask for Help

This is hard for many people to do. Some take it as a sign of their own weakness, but you wouldn't judge a friend as weak if they asked for your help. It's not weak at all. It's human. Talk with your support system about the help you need and how hard it is for you to ask for it. And I'm sure you'll be just as happy to help someone else when you're feeling well enough.

209 Remember I-Statements

If you are upset with a friend or family member, remember I-statements. For example, "I felt hurt when I told you I was not feeling well enough to go out, and it seemed that you didn't believe me. You said that I looked fine, but I really did not feel well."

210 Clearly Communicate Your Needs

Be clear and assertive. Tell your friends and family your exact needs. These may be obvious to you, but not to them. For this reason, it is better not to assume. For example, "I need you to believe me when I say I don't feel well. Please come with me to a support group so you can see I'm not the only one who looks well but doesn't feel well."

211 Be Realistic about Strengths and Limitations

We can't force people to be more supportive, attentive, or helpful. Some people will not be able to give you what you need. Learn people's strengths and limitations. For example, some people are wonderful when you need a good laugh, but aren't the best listeners when you need to express your feelings.

212 Invite a Loved One to a Support Group

Hearing the experiences of others is one of the best ways for people without lupus to gain an understanding of life with lupus. Some people invite loved ones to their first meeting for extra support. Others wait until they feel comfortable in the group before inviting anyone. You can also invite them to join online groups.

213 Invite Your Loved Ones to a Lupus Education Event

Invite your loved ones to lupus-related education events. They will learn a lot about lupus and establish a connection to the lupus community.

214 Acknowledge Support from Loved Ones

If they attend a support group or lupus education event, or if they support you in any other way, thank them. Showing appreciation helps strengthen the relationship and lets them know that they are supporting you in a much-needed way.

215 Explain Fatigue and Pain

It is easier for people without lupus to imagine what fatigue and pains feel like if reminded how they feel when they are in bed with a bad cold or the flu. Their body hurts and aches all over. They might feel sharp pain in their joints. Their body feels lifeless, heavy, and drained of all its energy. It's hard to get out of bed or do the smallest thing.

216 Come Up with Other Comparisons

Other people with lupus describe the pain and fatigue as feeling like they ran a marathon. Some say the fatigue feels like a ton of bricks holding them down. Try to think of other examples that can help the people in your life understand what these common lupus symptoms feel like. And, certainly, recommend that they download and read Christine Miserandino's *The Spoon Theory*—this easy-to-understand explanation of energy and fatigue really helps non-lupus people "get it."

217 Be Specific about the Pain

Be specific about pain because pain can mean a lot of things and take many forms. Explain if it is a dull pain, a sharp pain, and so on, and exactly where the pain is located. For example, specify if it is an all-over body ache, if it's in certain joints, in the muscles, all of these, or something else.

218 Explain Mood Changes Due to Medication or Pain

It is important to let your loved ones know the things that can negatively impact your mood, like steroids or pain. Also explain to them what help you need from them, and how you want them to respond in these situations.

219 Possible Reasons for Lack of Support

When someone is not supportive, it is often more about them than you— their being in denial that someone they love has an illness; their not knowing how to respond; their lack of communication skills. Knowing this can help you cope with their behavior, though it won't make things any less difficult.

220 Grieve Unsupportive People

I encourage you to seek comfort about unsupportive loved ones because this can be a serious loss. Share your feelings with your support system. You will quickly find that you are far from alone in these experiences.

221 Limit Communication with Unsupportive or Toxic People

You do not have to endure unsupportive or toxic behavior. When attempts at repairing a relationship do not work, limit interactions with people you feel are toxic or unhealthy to be around.

222 Ask for Help with Communication

If you are finding it difficult to communicate effectively, including limiting interactions to avoid toxic or unhealthy behavior, seek help from others with lupus to learn what strategies have worked well for them. Also consider speaking with a therapist about communicating with friends and family.

223 Support for Friends and Family

Lupus impacts the people who love you. They will need support, too. Lupus support groups can be enough for some, but others who provide a high level of caregiving may need to attend a caregiver support group. Your local lupus organization, support group members, hospital social workers, or doctors might know of some local resources.

Maintaining a Social Life

224 Be Realistic about Your Capabilities

Being realistic about what you can and cannot do because of lupus can be hard. You might not be able to socialize in the same ways you did pre-lupus. You may have to change or modify your habits according to your abilities, energy, and needs. If this is particularly upsetting for you, share this with your support system.

225 Know Your Types of Friends

Naturally, it will be easier to communicate and make plans with your friends with lupus or chronic illness since there is a shared understanding of issues such as flares, fatigue, and pain. With your other friends, however, you might need to communicate differently. You might have to explain how you feel, your abilities, and your needs. Knowing these differences can help you to manage your expectations of people without lupus or chronic illness.

226 Find a Middle Ground

Don't isolate yourself because of lupus. Find a middle ground that allows you to socialize comfortably. For example, you might not stay out late dancing, but perhaps you can go to dinner with friends, and maybe you can get in a dance or two before heading home. Or maybe you invite people to your place instead of going out.

227 Saying "No" or Canceling Plans

If you decline an invitation or have to cancel plans at the last minute, let your friends and family know that you are as upset and disappointed as they are. Assure them that it is not personal and has everything to do with how you are feeling.

228 Ask Friends to Ask You to Go Out

Let your loved ones know that even if you must say no or cancel plans, it doesn't mean that you are not interested. Let them know that an easy way to keep connected and be inclusive is to continue to invite you out and be understanding if you can't go. Explain that when they ask, it lets you know they haven't forgotten about you.

229 Get Good Rest

If you plan on attending an event, be sure to prepare. You may need to schedule a day both before and after the event to rest.

Managing Busy Holidays

230 Plan for the Holidays

Plan well in advance for the holidays because they arrive before you know it. Manage your energy by leaving enough space between tasks, such as buying or making gifts, food shopping, baking and cooking, traveling, attending parties, and so on. If you are hosting, try making it a potluck.

231 Coping with the Holidays

Stay in touch with how you feel physically and emotionally and then address any rising stress. It is extra important to implement communication skills, energy management, and stress reduction strategies during this time. Saying "No" is important: Don't take on too much. But do take extra special care of yourself. You don't want to get sick from the stress of the holidays.

232 Gift Giving and the Holidays

Gift giving, especially during the holidays, can be difficult for people with lupus, especially for anyone on a fixed income like SSI/SSDI. Shop all year round when you find sales. Stick to a budget. Consider making simple gifts, or writing poetry or heartfelt cards. Secret-gift exchanges or grab bags can help cut costs.

Romantic Relationships

Dating

233 Ask Yourself if You Are Ready to Date

Adjusting to and coming to terms with a life with lupus often require a lot of emotional energy. Ask yourself if you have the emotional energy to deal with dating as well. You'll know when you are ready.

234 Ready to Date? Go for It!

Lupus and dating might seem tricky, but it is not only possible, it's actually common. Recognize that you can date if you have lupus. If dating is something you feel ready to do, go for it!

235 Telling Your Date about Lupus

There is no perfect time to tell the person you are dating about lupus. If you hope to be with someone for the long term, they should know. You should share this information when you feel comfortable. Some people are upfront from the beginning. Others prefer to see if mutual feelings develop first.

236 Explain Lupus

When you do share the fact that you have lupus, explain what it is and clear up any concerns the other person might have. For example, they may want to know if it is life threatening, contagious, or degenerative.

237 Fatigue and Dating

Just as you would with any other social interaction, think ahead about your energy needs. Rest up if you have a long night ahead of you. Or choose to do something more low key.

238 Dealing with Rejection

Rejection is hard. And if you find that you were rejected because someone couldn't handle your condition, that hurts. You need someone who can be there for you in both easy and challenging times.

239 Finding the Right Person

The right person for you will not see lupus as a burden or run away in fear. The right person will care for you and want to be there for you, just as you want to be there for them in any way you can. The right person will know that, even though lupus impacts every part of your life, you are more than lupus. This person exists. Don't settle for someone who isn't supportive.

240 Find Balance

Try to find a good balance between communicating your needs, considering your partner's needs, and remembering that you *and* your relationship are much more than lupus. If you are in a serious relationship, it's never too early to see a couples' therapist. The sessions can help you build a strong foundation with good communication skills.

241 Encourage Honesty

If your partner does a lot of caregiving, they will need support, too. Encourage your partner to let you know when they are tired, need to recharge, or need support. Without support, resentment can build and put a strain on your relationship. But with the right support, a strong, happy, healthy relationship is possible.

242 Include Your Partner

Include your partner in lupus-related activities and be open about your health status. They care about you and want to be involved.

243 Take Care of Yourself

Taking care of yourself is not only important for your own quality of life, but for your partner and loved one's. They care about you, want you to live your best life with lupus, and want to share that life with you. You are loved and you matter.

Sex

244 Address a Low Sex Drive

Fatigue, depression, body image concerns, muscle and joint pain, hormone levels, and medication side effects could each lead to decreased sex drive. Talk with your doctor. They will help you pinpoint the cause and come up with a solution, such as adjusting medication or suggesting pain medication to take before sex.

245 Address Pain and Fatigue

If you experience muscle and joint pain during sex, try different positions until you find one that feels comfortable. Try having sex during a time of day when pain and fatigue are typically lowest. A warm bath before sex might be a soothing antidote.

246 Get Treatment for Gynecological Problems and Erectile Dysfunction

Gynecological problems could include vaginal dryness, irregular or heavy periods, vaginal sores, and painful orgasms. Erectile dysfunction can be caused by a medication side effect or a change in hormone levels due to lupus. If you are experiencing any of these, discuss them with your doctor to get appropriate medical treatment.

247 Help for Vaginal Dryness

Experiment with water-based lubricants, longer foreplay, and masturbation. Your doctor might be able to determine the cause or suggest other options.

248 Managing Raynaud's Phenomenon in the Bedroom

If you have pain in your hands and feet during sex due to Raynaud's phenomenon, try lying on your back. It puts less pressure on your extremities. Also, make sure the room is not too cold. Wear socks if you need to.

249 Let Your Partner Know Less Sex Is Not Their Fault

Communicate honestly with your partner about the challenges of having sex. This will help prevent them from taking your decreased drive personally. Communication will also help you explore alternatives to intercourse.

250 Tell Your Partner, It's Okay to Initiate Sexual Intimacy

Let your partner know that it's okay to initiate sexual intimacy. Otherwise, some partners may avoid intimacy out of fear of hurting you. This could generate resentment in you both, with each assuming the other is not interested.

251 Be Sexually Creative with Your Partner

If intercourse is too much for you right now, there are many other ways to experience sexual intimacy. You can try foreplay only, mutual masturbation, sex toys, and massage. Finding new and creative solutions can also strengthen your bond.

Family Planning

252 Lupus Medication and Infertility

Regardless of sex or gender, if having a family is important to you, speak with your doctor about your medications. Find out if infertility is a possible side effect.

253 Grieve Infertility

Sometimes, there is no alternative to using medication that might cause infertility. For many people, this is a terrible loss. Find support to help you cope with the grief.

254 Speak with Your Rheumatologist about Family Planning

Speak with your rheumatologist before trying to conceive. You need to work with your doctor to stay flare free for several months before conceiving. This greatly decreases chances of serious complications for both you and the baby. Your doctor also needs to evaluate your medication—some are unsafe for pregnancy.

255 See a High-Risk Obstetrician

People with lupus can have successful pregnancies and deliver healthy babies, but still need to be monitored for complications like preterm birth and pre-eclampsia. Ask your rheumatologist, gynecologist, support group peers, or lupus organization for recommendations for a high-risk obstetrician. And the best time to do this is *before* becoming pregnant.

256 Keep All Appointments with Your Rheumatologist and Obstetrician

You should be keeping all your appointments anyway, but, given lupus-related pregnancy risks, it is critically important that you and the baby's health status are monitored and assessed regularly. You will likely see your rheumatologist at least once a trimester, if not more, and your obstetrician more often than that.

257 Is It a Flare or Pregnancy?

If you become pregnant after working with your rheumatologist to stabilize lupus, it is unusual to have a flare during pregnancy. However, it is still important to determine if certain symptoms, such as fatigue, swelling joints, water retention, or hair loss, are from pregnancy or lupus. If you are experiencing these symptoms, let your rheumatologist know.

258 See Your Rheumatologist after Delivery

After you give birth, your body will go through many changes. It's important to see your rheumatologist after birth to monitor any lupus symptoms.

259 To Breastfeed or Not to Breastfeed?

Speak with your rheumatologist about your medication and breastfeeding. There are some medications that you cannot be on while breastfeeding because they would be passed to the baby. If you have to be on these medications, then you cannot breastfeed.

260 Lupus and Birth Control Pills

There is concern that hormone levels in some birth control pills could lead to higher risks of flares or blood clots. Different types of pills contain different levels and types of hormones. And different people with lupus present with different risk factors. So, while birth control pills might not be safe for one person, they could be safe for another. Speak to your rheumatologist about the best birth control method for you.

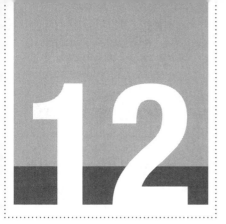

Parenting

261 Tell Your Children

Don't hide lupus from your children. They will pick up on mood, energy, and behavior changes. If you need help, ask others in your support system how they told their children about lupus. Find a book that you like that deals with talking to children about a parent's illness. A psychotherapist or a doctor with good bedside manner can also help answer medical questions your child has.

262 Explain Lupus in Simple Terms to Young Children

Explain lupus in simple, age-appropriate terms and concepts. Explain that it causes your body to hurt and makes you very tired, which is why you can't play with them sometimes and need to lie down a lot. It is caused by your body being confused and is not their fault in any way.

263 Explain Lupus to Preteens and Teens

Preteens and teens will be able to understand more and in more sophisticated language. You'll be able to explain your experience with lupus in greater detail—like what flares are and what causes them, and why you sometimes seem forgetful or unfocused. Explain only what is necessary—especially those symptoms that most affect your ability to function as a parent—and what will cause the least worry.

264 Allow Your Children to Ask Tough Questions

Your children need to know that they can ask you anything. Reassure them. Some might not have questions right now, but they should know that you are always there to answer any that might arise later.

265 Don't Ignore Behavior Changes

Take note if your child's behavior changes—if they become angry or withdrawn, for instance. Speak with them, their teachers, and, if necessary, a psychotherapist. They could be responding to their feelings and fears about lupus or to another challenge in life.

266 Don't Make Promises You Can't Keep

Life with lupus is often a "definite maybe" since you don't know how you will feel day to day. There will be times, for instance, that you might miss a school event. Let your child know ahead of time that you very much want to attend, that you will do your best to be there, but you might not feel well that day. This type of honest communication will help prevent broken promises.

267 If You Have to Cancel Plans with Your Children

If you have to cancel plans, talk openly with your children, hear their disappointment, and validate their feelings. Explore ways you can make it up to them when you feel better.

268 Addressing Concerns about Death

Let your kids speak openly about their fears. Let them know that most people with lupus live a normal life span. But be careful that you never say or imply that you will never die. Focus on what you are doing to stay as healthy as possible for as long as possible.

269 Continue the Conversation

You will need to keep communication open and honest with your children. Telling them about lupus isn't a one-time event. Depending on age, some children will not understand the persistent, off-and-on nature of chronic illness. They will need to know when you are having good days and not-so-good days, and what that means for them.

270 Spend Quality Time with Your Children

A lot of parents with lupus feel guilty about not spending as much time with their kids as they would like. The quality of the time you spend with your kids matters much more than the amount. Being a good listener and being engaged and involved in your moments together—that's what is invaluable, even if those moments are fewer than desired.

271 Seek Out Other Parents with Chronic Illness

Connecting with other parents with chronic illness will help you feel less guilty, less alone, and more supported. Hearing their experiences will help normalize yours. Plus, it's a great way to share useful ideas and information.

272 Find Out How Other Parents Solve Problems

You will face the challenges of not having enough energy to spend time with your children or getting things done around the house. But don't reinvent the wheel. Before wracking your brain, first find out what other parents are doing to solve these problems---maybe you can adapt their fixes to your life.

273 When Planning for a Flare, Include Your Family

Planning for a flare is especially important if you have children to care for. It's helpful to write down what each family member's role will be when you have a flare and talk with them about it before a flare occurs. Figure out who will be in charge of what and who will delegate when you are not feeling well.

274 Balancing Children's Chores

Kids commonly do chores. In a lupus household, parents sometimes need their kids to do even more. Do the best you can to balance their work and play.

275 Get Help

If it's within your budget, hire a babysitter to help you with childcare and chores even when you are home. Teenage babysitters, family members, or family friends are often affordable and maybe even free. Loved ones can help in other ways, too. For example, maybe someone could bring over dinner once or twice a week or help with laundry.

276 Make Yourself a Priority

It may sound counterintuitive, but the best way to care for your family is to take care of yourself. If you don't manage your energy, stress levels, and health, eventually this will catch up with you. Making yourself a priority is good for everyone.

277 Give Yourself Credit

Parents with lupus can be hard on themselves for not being able to do all the things they want to do with their children. Remember, no one's family life is ideal. You are doing the best you can. Managing lupus is a big job and the greatest gift you can give to your family.

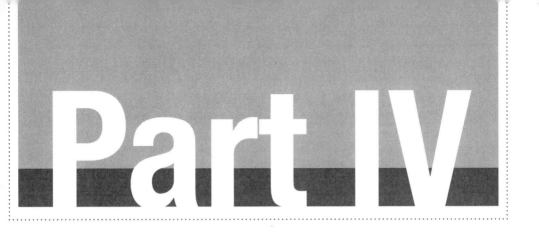

Part IV

Navigating the World with Lupus

13 Advance Directives

278 Complete Advance Directives

Advanced directives are written documents that provide instructions for your healthcare providers and loved ones should you become incapacitated. Every adult should have advance directives regardless of age or health status.

279 Make Sure Your Health Care Wishes Are Communicated

Completing these forms will help ensure your wishes are respected in the event that you can't make them clear yourself. It will also help your family struggle less with figuring out the appropriate choices to make.

280 Look Up Advance Directives by State

There are two main types of advance directives. For the first, a living will, you list end-of-life medical choices. With the second, a durable power of attorney for health care, you choose someone to make health care decisions for you should you be too incapacitated to communicate---this person is called a health care proxy It is wise to have both documents. Each state has its own laws concerning advance directives.

281 Think about Future Health Care Choices

These are difficult choices to make, which is why they are often avoided. You need to decide how you want your doctors and family to proceed with your health care when you are incapacitated or unable to make decisions for yourself—being under anesthesia, in a coma, or having severe dementia, for example. Choices for end-of-life care include organ donation; "do not resuscitate" orders; whether you want a ventilator or a breathing machine, dialysis, a feeding tube, and so on. Communicate your choices to your loved ones so they are aware of your wishes, and include them in your living will and durable power of attorney for health care.

282 Provide Copies to Your Doctors and Loved Ones

If no one knows you have these documents, it's as if you don't have them. Be sure to share and review them with your trusted loved ones and your doctors.

283 Update Your Advance Directives

Remember to update your advance directives whenever necessary. Including if your contact information changes, or if you have changed your mind about a future health care choice or who you want your proxy to be. All previous copies need to be destroyed and new copies distributed.

284 Choose Your Health Care Proxy Wisely

Choose someone you trust, who doesn't live too far away and seems to have a real understanding of both your health care wishes and how lupus affects you. Have a discussion with your proxy to be sure they are comfortable with this role. If there is no one you'd choose as your proxy, it is still important to document your health care wishes. Share these with your health care providers and let them know you did not choose anyone to be your proxy.

285 Prepare a Last Will and Testament and Financial Power of Attorney

Preparing a last will and testament is another one of those things we all know we should do but tend to delay. When you do prepare a will, consider also appointing a financial power of attorney who will have control over your finances should you become incapacitated. This is a very powerful document so you must choose very carefully. Also, speak with your financial institutions when you complete this document—they will likely want a copy.

286 Seek Legal Help

You can find almost all of these forms online for free, but it is wise to seek legal help for a last will and testament and financial power of attorney. If you cannot afford legal help, seek assistance from a legal aid program, a local law school, or your state's bar association.

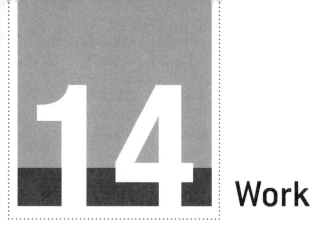

Work

287 Consider Financial, Emotional, and Physical Needs

Whether you are job searching, changing fields, or reinventing yourself, think about what kind of work meets your financial, emotional, and physical needs. Some jobs are physically demanding or require long hours, for example. Most situations are not 100% ideal, so weigh the pros and cons for each one and choose what best meets your criteria.

288 Continue to Prioritize Your Health

Don't forget to manage your energy at work. Prioritize tasks. Try not to overwork. Take short breaks by stretching your legs or any part of your body that might feel stiff. These are the types of little things that can have long-term benefits.

289 Telling Your Employer about Lupus

There's no definitive answer about whether and when you should tell your employer about lupus. The rule of thumb is to share on an as-needed basis, and not to share more information than necessary.

290 Assess Your Work Environment

Take stock of your workplace. What is your boss's personality like? What is the office culture? Is there a human resources department to help keep your information private? These factors could impact your willingness to disclose that you have lupus.

291 Accommodations in the Workplace

Sometimes you have to ask for accommodations in order to continue to work. The Americans with Disabilities Act (ADA) allows employees to request reasonable accommodations from their employer. If you need them, ask for them, but the ADA does not apply to all employers. Contact the Job Accommodation Network for more information.

292 How to Request an Accommodation

Be specific about what accommodations you need. Explain how your performance and attendance are impacted by current limitations, and how the accommodations will help you to continue working and be productive. Put the request in writing so that you have proof of your request, and review it with your employer during a face-to-face meeting. Seeing and hearing you only serves to humanize your request.

293 Requesting Time Off

A common accommodation to help manage flares and medical appointments is having a flexible schedule and being able to take necessary time off. Many employees are covered under the Family and Medical Leave Act (FMLA), which protects their jobs when they need to take extended or periodic time off for themselves or to take care of a loved one. Speak with your employer about your scheduling needs.

294 Types of Accommodations

Think outside the box about your request. Accommodations can be about your schedule, prioritizing or changing job duties, placing light shields over fluorescent bulbs and computer screens, taking more frequent and/or longer breaks, having an ergonomic chair and workspace, and so on. Be open to suggestions from your employer, as well.

295 Work from Home

Working from home—also called working remotely or telecommuting—could be a solution to your employment challenges. Some work-at-home jobs are 100% home based. Others are part at-home, part in-office. Red-flag alert: Beware of work-at-home scams that ask you to pay a fee for anything. When in doubt, search online for company reviews and, certainly, read up on the many types of home-based schemes out there. Simply search "work-at-home scams"; several good and useful websites will pop right up.

296 Consider Other Employment Alternatives

Some people move from a traditional work environment into freelance work or self-employment. These alternatives offer them the advantage of schedule flexibility, which helps with managing lupus symptoms. Other people opt to reduce their hours to part time if their employer is agreeable and the money makes sense.

297 When to Stop Working

If lupus is interfering with your ability to work, and working from home or workplace accommodations are not helpful enough, it might be time to stop working altogether, at least temporarily. Some people may need to take a short-term leave to recover from surgery, for example, with the intention of returning to work.

Plan Ahead

Try to think ahead about what you would do to pay your bills if you had to stop working. You might need to start saving money, consider the possibility of living with a family member or getting a roommate, or exploring whether it would be feasible to rely on your partner's income. Income from disability is another option.

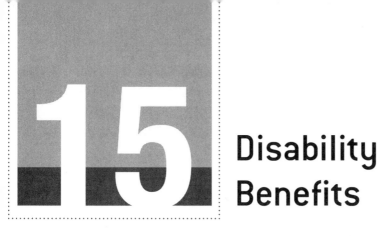

Disability Benefits

299 Short-Term Disability Benefits from Your State

Contact your state's Department of Labor to find out about short-term disability for a temporary, non-work-related illness. You may be eligible if you have an illness, an injury, or are unable to work because of pregnancy or complications from childbirth.

300 Short- and Long-Term Disability Insurance through Your Employer

These are available through your employer from a private insurance company. Short-term disability insurance is different than what is available from the state. Long-term disability insurance could possibly be paid out to you for the rest of your life should you become permanently disabled. Check with your employer to find out if these are offered, and about eligibility and enrollment.

301 Financial Planning

You will receive less income on disability than from employment earnings, so it's important to examine your expenses and budget according to estimated disability income, not employment earnings. If you are on disability and married, be sure that you are named a beneficiary on your spouse's bank and retirement accounts as well as last will and testament. In this way, your access to these funds is protected should the worst happen to your loved one.

302 Applying for SSI/SSDI

If you become permanently disabled, you can apply for disability through the federal government. Eligibility for Social Security Disability Insurance (SSDI) depends on the amount and length of your work history. People without enough work history could be eligible for Supplemental Security Income (SSI) instead.

303 Get a Lawyer

It is hard to get approved for SSI or SSDI. I strongly suggest using a disability attorney and not going through the Social Security Administration (SSA) on your own. Your local lupus organization and/or support group should be able to recommend a good disability lawyer.

304 Retirement or SSDI?

If you are near retirement age, speak with your lawyer or the Social Security Administration about the advantages of applying for retirement instead of disability. Some people will choose to apply for retirement benefits if they need money quickly because approval is based on age, not on proving that you have a disability. Others will decide that applying for disability is better than applying for early retirement since the latter means accepting a reduced monthly Social Security benefit. In some cases, you can get both. Yes, it's complicated, and all the more reason to enlist the assistance of a disability lawyer.

305 Explain How Lupus Prevents You from Working

It is important to communicate clearly about how lupus has interfered with your ability to work when speaking with your lawyer, anyone from the SSA (including their doctors), the state about short-term disability, or your disability insurers. Having lupus does not automatically qualify you for disability.

306 Applying for SSDI after Being Approved for Long-Term Disability

Check with your long-term disability insurance company about their policy for applying for SSDI. It is likely that they will require you to apply for SSDI and then reduce the amount they pay you based on your SSDI payment. They might urge you to use their lawyer to help you apply, but their interests, not yours, are their priority. Get your own lawyer.

307 Affording a Lawyer for SSI/SSDI

Typically, lawyers charge a percentage based on the back money you are awarded once you are approved for SSI/SSDI. They cannot charge more than 25% or $6,000 (subject to change according to SSA guidelines). For example, if you apply for disability on December 1 of this year and get approved the following December, your payments might start from the day you applied, not the day you were approved, and you will get back money for that year.

308 Get Your Medical Paperwork in Order

Before you see a lawyer, get your paperwork in order. This includes medical paperwork from your doctors, hospital stays, and emergency room visits. Go as far back as possible relevant to when your conditions started. Also, make a list of your current prescriptions and document the side effects you experience with each medication.

309 Include Every Condition

For your SSI/SSDI application, you should include information about every condition, from lupus to migraines and high blood pressure to depression. Everything counts. Do not leave anything out.

310 Get Your Work History Together

Document your work and income history. This should include where you worked, for how long, what your job responsibilities were, and your income. Be able to explain how your conditions prevent you from performing those responsibilities.

311 Get Support from Your Doctors

Before you apply for disability, it's important to speak with your doctors about whether they support your application. It's helpful to have their support because they will have to state, in required documentation, whether or not they believe you can work. If you don't have their support, you can still apply if you believe you cannot work, especially if you are working with a lawyer.

312 The Benefit of Consistent Medical Care

The longer you have been with a doctor, the better they know you and how your conditions impact your life and the better they can support your claim that you can no longer work. Do your best to have consistent medical care. But if that hasn't been possible for any reason, you should still apply for disability.

313 Know the Date of Disability versus the Date of Application

When you apply for disability of any kind, know that there is a difference between the date you became unable to work versus the date you are applying. If you cannot pinpoint an exact date, estimate when you became disabled. The date you became disabled and unable to work could impact how much back pay you get, or even if you get approved. Ideally, you'd be able to show that you were disabled or will be disabled for 12 months or more. To get a full year of pay prior to the application date, a person applying for SSDI (not SSI) has to show that they were disabled at least 17 months before applying. Because this can be confusing, it's best to speak with your lawyer about these details.

314 Find Out about Exclusions

Always read the fine print to find out the reasons you can be refused disability benefits through private insurance companies. These are called exclusions. In addition, there might be a waiting period for pre-existing conditions like lupus.

315 Appeal a Denial

If you enroll in a disability insurance plan and get denied, find out why and appeal. The same goes for federal disability. Also, if you applied for SSI/SSDI without a lawyer, and need to appeal, it's not too late. You can still engage a disability lawyer to help you appeal for both government and private benefits.

316 Disability Insurance for Self-Employed People and Freelancers

If you are self-employed, it may be harder—but not impossible—to find insurance that allows for pre-existing conditions. If you freelance, check with the Freelancer's Union to find out if you can enroll in what they offer.

317 Before Returning to Work...

Volunteering is one way to figure out whether you are able to work without involving the SSA or your insurer. But earning over a certain amount could impact your disability and health benefits. Because of this, speak to your insurer, SSA, and/or a lawyer before returning to work to find out how working could interfere with your benefits and how to avoid this interference when returning to work

318 Learn about Vocational Rehabilitation Programs

If you decide to try going back to work, even part time, the SSA has a Ticket-to-Work program that can help with training and job placement. Contact them for more information. If you are not on disability through SSA, you can contact your state's vocational rehabilitation office for assistance.

319 Learn about Expedited Reinstatement

If you go back to work and it doesn't pan out, you don't necessarily have to start the application for SSI/SSDI all over again. As of this writing, there is something called expedited reinstatement. Before you start working, discuss this with the SSA. Also, talk to your disability insurer about the process for getting disability insurance reinstated, but do so before you start working.

16 Higher Education

320 Include Your Doctors

Let your doctors know you are headed for college, and that you might need them to provide the school with documentation showing you have a chronic illness. Ask your doctors for advice about managing lupus as a college student. Make sure you get prescription refills if the school is far away. Get a copy of your health records to take with you. Remember to schedule your next appointment.

321 Decide Where You Will Get Medical Care

If you go to school far from home, you need to decide if you will continue seeing the same rheumatologist or see one near school. The advantage of keeping your current doctor is that you have a history with them. The advantage of seeing someone near you is that you have access to a rheumatologist when you need one and in emergencies. You may still be able to see your current rheumatologist when you visit home, depending on what your insurance allows.

322 Connect with the Office of Disability Services

People with lupus may not consider themselves disabled, so they might not think to contact their school's disability services office (sometimes referred to by other names like Office of Special Services or Accessibility Services). Contact them anyway. Once you are connected, the office will be there to advocate for you if you fall behind and to help you obtain any necessary accommodations. You should also make sure to inquire about their other services and resources.

323 Check Out the College Health Center

Familiarize yourself with the college health center. Find out what services they provide. Some health centers have full medical staff, and others have very limited services. Either way, ask if they have ever had any patients with lupus and how they might be able to help you while you are at school. Find out if they have late hours or 24-hour coverage and note their contact information.

324 Take Care of Yourself

In order to do well and stay in school, your health is a priority. Be sure to keep your medical appointments, take your medication as prescribed, practice self-care by getting enough rest, and implement stress management, time management, and organization techniques. Always check with your doctor or pharmacist about prescription and alcohol interactions.

325 Be Careful with Your Course Load

Don't take on too many courses at once. It's better to take longer to graduate than to get sick from stress, fall behind, or be forced to take time off.

326 Schedule Rest Times

It's easy to lose track of time when you are busy. To help make sure that you get enough rest each day, schedule breaks and naps into your daily schedule.

327 Record Lectures

With your professor's permission, make audio recordings of lectures to help you remember the material later—especially if you experience lupus fog. If you have to miss class, perhaps a friend can record the class for you.

328 Be Informed about Financial Aid Policies

If you have to withdraw from a class, your financial aid could be impacted. Speak with someone at your school's financial aid office at the start of the semester to learn about this.

329 Officially Drop a Course

Sometimes people feel so overwhelmed, anxious, or embarrassed about falling behind in school because of lupus that they stop attending class and don't officially withdraw. If you have to withdraw, first contact the disabilities office to see if they can help. If they can't, officially drop the course or courses. Not showing up for class could result in a failing grade and interfere with your overall G.P.A., enrollment, scholarships, and financial aid.

330 Communicate with Professors

Even if you are connected with the disabilities office, it is important to let your professors know of any challenges you face so you can negotiate a solution. Let them know you are connected with the disabilities office and request tolerance should you be sidelined by illness. Most will tend to be more flexible if they are kept in the loop.

331 Have a Support System in Place

It may be hard at first, but it is smart to let a good friend or two know that you have lupus and what to do in case of an emergency. They are the ones who can call your family, communicate with professors, and help communicate with medical staff if you have to go to the ER.

332 Educate Friends and Others

If you are comfortable talking about lupus publicly, educate your friends and other students. Find out if there's a local lupus organization nearby that can give a presentation in your dorm, for example. Or give your own.

333 Find Support for Lupus

Join a student club for people with chronic illness, if one exists on campus—or start one yourself. Find out if there are lupus support groups nearby that you can attend.

334 Find Balance

The same self-care, energy management, and communication practices for socializing discussed earlier apply to college students as well. College is a balancing act between prioritizing your health, managing your coursework, and socializing. You won't be able to do all the socializing you want. But you can do a lot without giving up self-care.

Traveling

335 Travel When Feeling Okay

If you are in the middle of a flare or experiencing any kind of illness, don't travel. In many cases, your body won't let you anyway, but it's an important caveat for those of us who are very stubborn or determined. Traveling is stressful and will only make you feel worse.

336 Talk with Your Doctor

Talk to your rheumatologist and other doctors about your trip early in the planning process—at least 4 to 10 weeks in advance. Ask for advice about traveling with lupus, including tips for flying. Ask for a signed letter that lists all your medical conditions and medication.

337 What to Do if You Lose Your Medication

Ask your doctor what to do if you lose your medication while traveling. They might provide you with extra prescriptions.

338 Pack Extra Medication

Ask for extra medication in case of a flare. Keep your supply of extra medication in a different location in case you lose the other supply. Fill your prescription before you leave, and be sure you have enough for when you get back. Be prepared with over-the-counter medications. You might need them for allergies (antihistamines), upset stomach (antacids), or diarrhea (anti-diarrhea), for example.

339 Traveling with a Suppressed Immune System

People with lupus tend to be at greater risk for infection because their medication suppresses their immune system. Ask your rheumatologist what you should do to protect yourself against infection when traveling. They might prescribe antibiotics to take during your travels.

340 Find Out about Vaccinations

Find out about any vaccinations you need if you are traveling internationally. If you need them, ask your rheumatologist if they are safe for you. If they are not, you will need to change plans and travel elsewhere or look into getting a medical exemption letter. If you choose the latter course, just make sure to discuss what your risks are without the vaccinations. Consider seeing a travel medicine specialist.

341 Consider Travel Insurance

If you can afford it, buy travel insurance in case you get sick and have to cancel plans. The extra cost could end up saving you money if you are unable to make the trip. Be sure to read the fine print and understand what is not covered under the insurance plan. Check if it covers pre-existing conditions and travel costs such as tickets and hotel.

342 Plan for Medical Care

If you have a medical need like dialysis that you cannot skip while you are away, you need to find reliable medical care. Speak with a social worker at your hospital, your doctor, or ask your local disease organization for help with this. Be sure that the medical facility you choose has a solid reputation.

343 Check Health Insurance Coverage

Call your health insurer and find out what you are covered for both out of state and internationally. For example, does your insurance cover a rheumatologist, emergency care, or other medical needs like dialysis?

344 Plan for an Emergency

Speak with your rheumatologist to develop a plan in the event of an emergency. Locate a good rheumatologist and quality medical center near your travel destination. Find out if there is a local lupus organization. Keep this information in an easy-to-find place, along with a copy of that signed letter from your doctor.

345 Get Ready Far in Advance

Do your best to start planning as far in advance as possible— 4 to 10 weeks depending on your situation. Pace yourself with every step of the planning process, including packing, notifying your post office and newspaper delivery, making arrangements for your pet, and so on. Waiting until the last minute will add stress to an already stressful process. Allow others to help you.

346 Let Your Travel Companions Know How to Help You

Make sure all of your travel companions know that you have a chronic illness early in the planning process. Let them know what to expect and how they can help you, including in the event of an emergency.

347 Make Rest a Priority

While on your trip, plan your days wisely and schedule them to include rest periods. This will help you manage your energy. Schedule time to rest before you leave for your trip and after you get back home. When sightseeing, consider what's easiest (e.g., tour buses instead of walking). A good travel guide — whether online or in book form—will identify those sites that are easiest to access.

348 Flying with Medication

Always try to bring your original prescription bottles when traveling. If you can't or you don't have the original bottles, bring a signed doctor's letter that lists your conditions and medication. For more information on flying with medication, contact the Transportation Security Administration.

349 Fly Comfortably

If you find the airport tiring, you can request a wheelchair. If it's within your budget, pick a seat on the plane with extra leg room. If you need sleeping pills for a long flight, remember to ask your doctor for a prescription. Don't forget a neck pillow and a blanket.

350 Drive Comfortably

Pack snacks, pillows, blankets, and any other items that will help you feel comfortable in the car. Take frequent breaks and rest stops. While they will lengthen travel time, hopefully they will make the drive less tiring.

351 Find an ADA-Compliant Hotel

If necessary, make sure your hotel is ADA compliant with a ramp, handicap parking, automatic doors, and working elevators. Ask for an ADA-compliant room with bars in the bathroom, a shower seat, and enough space for a wheelchair, for example.

Becoming a Lupus Advocate

Create Lupus Awareness

352 Get Involved in Your Local Lupus Organization

If there is a lupus organization in your area, consider getting involved. Learning more about lupus by attending their educational events will help you become a more informed advocate. Consider volunteering with them at health fairs or other events to help spread lupus awareness. Participate in their walks.

353 Share Information about Lupus

Share information about lupus in your community. Get free pamphlets about lupus from your local lupus organization or from the National Institute of Arthritis and Musculoskeletal and Skin Diseases (NIAMS). Leave these in public places you visit, such as doctor offices, local government offices (e.g., city council, community affairs), libraries, houses of worship, and so on, but always ask for permission.

354 Educate Your Doctors

The more doctors know about lupus, the better they will be at recognizing the symptoms. This will lead to quicker diagnosis. The Lupus Initiative is a program that exists to educate doctors and other medical professionals about lupus. Let everyone in your health care team know about this program and how to obtain its free material.

355 Organize Lupus Presentations

Help your community learn about lupus. Organize presentations at, your local school, library, or places of worship. If there is a lupus organization near you, ask them to present. Maybe your rheumatologist would be willing to give a brief talk. You, or someone else, could also share your story.

356 Raise Awareness on the Internet

Share stories and information on social media. Follow and interact with others talking about lupus. Use lupus-related hash tags (#lupus, #lupusawareness, #chronicillness, etc.). Also, consider blogging about your experience with lupus. This could be a therapeutic outlet for you and enlightening reading for others; and the feedback you get might be gratifying. Use your real name or be anonymous.

357 Tell Your Story in Pictures

Take pictures of what your daily life is like with lupus. Share them with your loved ones to help them better understand. For great examples of this, check out *Lupus through the Lens* online.

358 Start a Support Group

If there is no support group in your area, some lupus organizations—such as Molly's Fund—will train you in getting one up and running. This is your best option. Or look up information online about how to start and run a support group. Do a search for manuals. Contact a disease organization in your area that runs groups and ask for tips.

359 Take Part in a Lupus Walk

Walks are a great way to get friends and family involved in the lupus community. They also help raise awareness about lupus and raise money for lupus research. When you participate, you can choose to walk as much or as little as is comfortable.

Advocate for Health Care Policy and Funding

360 Sign Up for Advocacy Email Alerts

Sign up for advocacy-related email alerts from your local and national lupus organizations. They will keep you informed about important legislative advocacy issues and how to help. This might involve a letter, an e-mail, or a phone call to your local representative about health care policy or funding issues.

361 Contact Lupus Agencies

Call or e-mail these agencies directly and ask them how you can get more involved. This might lead to a more active role in lupus advocacy.

Help Make Medicine More Patient Centered

362 Get Involved in Participatory Medicine

Participatory medicine is a patient empowerment approach to health care. Advocates believe that health care should be patient-centric and not doctor-centric, especially when it comes to patient-education and health care decisions. Patient voices are a priority and health care providers should view patients as partners. To learn more, contact the Society for Participatory Medicine. Important topics to investigate are electronic health records (EHR) and health information privacy related to the Health Insurance Portability and Accountability Act (HIPAA).

363 Become an e-Patient

You are an e-patient if… you prioritize self-care; take an active role in your health care; use the Internet to find reliable information on lupus and its management; read and leave doctor reviews; join online support groups and communities; write blogs; use a phone app to help manage your health; sign online petitions and reach out to government officials via the Internet; or interact with others in the lupus community on social media, whether you choose to do so anonymously or not. This is part of participatory medicine and what is referred to as being an *e-patient*.

364 Participate in Patient-Centered Research

Historically, patients have not been allowed access to the research process. Usually, their connection to research is limited to being participants in clinical trials. The Patient-Centered Outcomes Research Institute (PCORI) provides opportunities for patients to propose research questions and involve themselves in every step of the research process, from beginning to end. You can apply to be part of one of their advisory panels and be involved in other ways.

Clinical Trials

365 Consider a Clinical Trial

One way to support the advancement of lupus research is to participate in a lupus clinical trial. These clinical trials are research studies that help us learn more about lupus and discover new, safer, and more effective treatments. People enrolled in trials that test medication, medical devices, or procedures receive very high-quality medical care and monitoring. There are also trials that do not require taking medication. Instead, some require blood or saliva samples, for example. There are even lupus trials that request participation from people without lupus.

Afterword

If I were to narrow down these hundreds of tips to the top three, I'd say: One, manage lupus with a rheumatologist you feel comfortable with. I know that finding a good rheumatologist will be easier for some than others, but don't give up. You need to stabilize your health before you can do much else. Two, learn about lupus. It's important to understand something that so significantly impacts your body and the rest of your life. Without this, it's hard to advocate for yourself as a patient or in your community. Three, find support.

If everything else in this book feels too hard right now, and you don't know where to begin, I strongly encourage you to do this one thing—find support. As you read, there are many ways to find support. And sometimes it is through your support system that you find the right doctor and other resources that you need.

Living with lupus without support can lead to isolation. Isolation will convince you that the negative thoughts you have about yourself are true, that you have somehow failed at life because of lupus, and that there is no hope. I have seen how support groups have helped many people begin to overcome this. Being believed and understood, hearing other stories, and sharing your own stories will help you realize that none of your struggles are in your imagination, that your feelings are valid, that there is hope, and that there are people who care about you and want you to do well.

Hearing and sharing stories is an important part of lupus support. Tell your story. Tell it as many times and in as many ways as you need to. Write it down. Say it aloud. Not only will it help you, but someone else will hear you and recognize themselves in your story. And that is a great and special gift.

Resources

*Some chapters do not include resources

Chapter 2 Getting the Medical Care You Need
American College of Rheumatology
Find a Member:
ww2.rheumatology.org/directory/geo.asp
404-633-3777
acr@rheumatology.org

Find a Health Center
U.S. Department of Health and Human Services
Health Resources and Services Administration
findahealthcenter.hrsa.gov/Search_HCC.aspx
*free or low-cost; you will not be turned down if you have no insurance

Free/Low Cost Clinic Finder
Partnership for Prescription Assistance
pparx.org/prescription_assistance_programs/free_clinic_finder

Freelancers Union
freelancersunion.org
800-856-9981
membership@freelancersunion.org

"Living With Cancer: The Good Patient Syndrome"
by Susan Gubar
The New York Times Blog, January 24, 2013
well.blogs.nytimes.com/2013/01/24/living-with-cancer-the-good-patient-syndrome

Health Insurance Marketplace
healthcare.gov
Individuals & Families: 800-318-2596/TTY: 855-889-4325
Small Businesses: 800-706-7893/TTY: 711

Medicare Rights Center
medicarerights.org
National Helpline: 800-333-4114
info@medicarerights.org

National Institute of Arthritis and Musculoskeletal and Skin Diseases (NIAMS)
niams.nih.gov/Health_Info/Lupus
Order free publications: catalog.niams.nih.gov
877-22-NIAMS (877-226-4267)
TTY: 301-565-2966
NIAMSinfo@mail.nih.gov

Patient Advocate Foundation
patientadvocate.org
800-532-5274

Prescription and Copay Assistance Programs
Partnership for Prescription Assistance
pparx.org
List of prescription savings cards:
pparx.org/prescription_assistance_programs/savings_cards

The HealthWell Foundation
healthwellfoundation.org
800-675-8416
grants@HealthWellFoundation.org
medication- and treatment-related financial assistance with coinsurance, copayments, and health care premiums; they have a program specifically for lupus

Lupus and Allied Diseases Association, Inc.
Prescription Resources
nolupus.org/prescription_resources0.aspx

Chapter 3 Medication and Treatment
Acupuncture and Lupus
"Acupuncture for SLE: Can it Work for You?"
Hospital for Special Surgery
hss.edu/conditions_acupuncture-for-sle-lupus.asp

American Massage Therapy Association
amtamassage.org
877-905-0577
info@amtamassage.org

"How to Read and Understand a Scientific Paper: A Step-by-Step Guide for Non-Scientists"
by Jennifer Raff
The Huffington Post, 6/18/2014
huffingtonpost.com/jennifer-raff/how-to-read-and-understand-a-scientific-paper_b_5501628.html

"New York Attorney General Targets Supplements at Major Retailers"
by Anahad O'Connor
The New York Times Blog, 2/3/2015
well.blogs.nytimes.com/2015/02/03/new-york-attorney-general-targets-supplements-at-major-retailers

National Center for Complementary and Integrative Health
U.S. Department of Health & Human Services
National Institutes of Health
nccih.nih.gov
888-644-6226
TTY: 866-464-3615

Sense About Science
senseaboutscience.org
"Making Sense of Chemical Stories"
senseaboutscience.org/pages/making-sense-of-chemical-stories.html
enquiries@senseaboutscience.org

Chapter 4 You Are Not Alone
Association for Death Education and Counseling
adec.org
847-509-0403
info@adec.org
resources about loss and grief, and help finding a grief counselor

Crisis Call Center
crisiscallcenter.org
Call anytime, 24/7/365
800-273-8255
or text ANSWER to 839863
offers help for crises like suicide prevention; intimate partner, child, and elder abuse; and substance abuse

Hospital for Special Surgery - National Lupus Programs

LupusLine®
Hospital for Special Surgery
hss.edu/lupus-programs.asp
866-375-1427
lupuslineprogram@hss.edu
*national, one-on-one peer telephone emotional support program for people with lupus

Charla de Lupus/Lupus Chat®
Hospital for Special Surgery
hss.edu/lupus-programs.asp
866-812-4494
charla@hss.edu
*national peer health support and education program for people with lupus and their families, in English and Spanish

LANtern® (Lupus Asian Network)
Hospital for Special Surgery
hss.edu/lupus-programs.asp
866-505-2253
tranm@hss.edu
*national bilingual support and education program serving Asian Americans with lupus and their families

National Alliance on Mental Illness
nami.org
Helpline: 800-950-6264
info@nami.org
helpline provides information on mental illness, along with referrals and resources

Chapter 7 Managing Stress

National Center for Complementary and Integrative Health
U.S. Department of Health & Human Services
National Institutes of Health
"Meditation: What You Need to Know"
nccih.nih.gov/health/meditation/overview.htm

The Greater Good Science Center
greatergood.berkeley.edu
510-642-2490
Greater@berkeley.edu
"Expanding Gratitude Project"
greatergood.berkeley.edu/expandinggratitude

The UC San Diego Center for Mindfulness
health.ucsd.edu/specialties/mindfulness
"Mindfulness Resources"
health.ucsd.edu/specialties/mindfulness/resources/Pages/
default.aspx

UCLA Mindful Awareness Research Center
marc.ucla.edu
310-206-7503
marcinfo@ucla.edu

Chapter 9 Lupus on the Outside

American Academy of Dermatology
aad.org
866-503-SKIN (7546)
International: 847-240-1280
"Sunscreen FAQs"
aad.org/media-resources/stats-and-facts/prevention-and-care/
sunscreen-faqs

"Psychosocial Dimensions of SLE: Implications for the Health Care Team"
by Nancy L Beckerman, Charles Auerbach, and Irene Blanco
Journal of Multidisciplinary Healthcare, 2011; 4: 63–72
ncbi.nlm.nih.gov/pmc/articles/PMC3093952

Chapter 10 Family and Friends

National Alliance for Caregiving
Resources for Caregivers
caregiving.org/resources
301-718-8444
info@caregiving.org

The Spoon Theory
by Christine Miserandino
butyoudontlooksick.com/articles/written-by-christine/
the-spoon-theory
available in English, Spanish, French, and Hebrew

Chapter 13 Advance Directives

Aging with Dignity
fivewishes.org
888-5WISHES (594-7437)
fivewishes@agingwithdignity.org
referred to as "the living will with a heart and soul"

National Healthcare Decisions Day (NHDD)
Advance Care Planning Resource
nhdd.org/public-resources#where-can-i-get-an-advance-directive

U.S. Living Will Registry
uslivingwillregistry.com
800-LIV-WILL (800-548-9455)
admin@uslivingwillregistry.com

Finding Free or Low Cost Legal Assistance

American Bar Association
americanbar.org
800-285-2221

Legal Services Corporation
"Find Legal Aid"
lsc.gov/find-legal-aid
202-295-1500

Chapter 14 Work

Job Accommodation Network
askjan.org
800-526-7234
TTY: 877-781-9403
"Accommodation and Compliance Series: Employees with Lupus"
askjan.org/media/Lupus.html
Vocational Rehabilitation Programs by State
askjan.org/cgi-win/TypeQuery.exe?902

The National Disability Rights Network
ndrn.org
202-408-9514
TTY: 220-408-9521
provides assistance with multiple issues for people with disabilities

United States Department of Justice
Civil Rights Division
Information and Technical Assistance on the Americans with
Disabilities Act
ada.gov
800-514-0301
TTY: 800-514-0383

United States Department of Labor Office of Disability Employment
Policy
dol.gov/odep
866-ODEP-DOL (633-7365)
877-TTY-5627 (877-889-5627)
odep@dol.gov

United States Department of Labor
Wage and Hour Division
"Family and Medical Leave Act"
dol.gov/whd/fmla
866-4USWAGE (866-487-9243)
TTY: 1-877-889-5627

Chapter 15 Disability Benefits

Disability.gov
disability.gov
resources for people with disabilities, their families, and caregivers

The United States Social Security Administration
ssa.gov
800-772-1213
TTY: 800-325-0778

Chapter 16 Higher Education

Lupus Inspiration Foundation for Excellence (L.I.F.E.) Scholarship
lifescholarship.org
life4lupuscholarship@gmail.com

Chapter 17 Traveling

Centers for Disease Control and Prevention
Traveler Information Center
wwwnc.cdc.gov/travel/page/traveler-information-center
"Obtaining Healthcare Abroad for the Ill Traveler"
wwwnc.cdc.gov/travel/yellowbook/2014/chapter-2-the-pre-
travel-consultation/obtaining-health-care-abroad-for-the-ill-traveler
Find a Clinic (travel medicine)
wwwnc.cdc.gov/travel/page/find-clinic

International Association for Medical Assistance to Travelers
iamat.org
716-754-4883

Transportation Security Administration
tsa.gov
866-289-9673
TSA-ContactCenter@tsa.dhs.gov
"TSA Travel Tips Tuesday - Traveling With Medication"
blog.tsa.gov/2013/09/tsa-travel-tips-tuesday-traveling-with.html
"Travelers with Disabilities and Medical Conditions"
tsa.gov/traveler-information/travelers-disabilities-
and-medical-conditions
TSA Cares Helpline
855-787-2227
provides help for travelers with disabilities and medical conditions

Chapter 18 Becoming a Lupus Advocate

Lupus through the Lens
lupuslens.wordpress.com
The S.L.E. Lupus Foundation community captured, in pictures, what it means to live with lupus

The Lupus Initiative
thelupusinitiative.org
404-633-3777
free resources for healthcare professionals and students to learn more about lupus

National Lupus Organizations and Directories

Alliance for Lupus Research
lupusresearch.org
800-867-1743
info@lupusresearch.org

Lupus Foundation of America
Find a chapter in the U.S.: lupus.org/chapters
International resources: lupus.org/resources/international-resources
202-349-1155
info@lupus.org

Lupus Research Institute
National Coalition Members:
lupusresearchinstitute.org/lupus-advocacy/lupus-national-coalition-members
212-812-9881
Lupus@LupusNY.org
The LRI's Coalition members are independent lupus organizations located in the U.S.

Molly's Fund
mollysfund.org/programs-services
503-775-3497
info@mollysfund.org
located in Oregon, but has an online support group, groups around the U.S., and a national support-group training program

Patient-Centered Medicine

e-Patient Dave
epatientdave.com
603-459-5119
dave@epatientdave.com

Office of the National Coordinator for Health Information Technology
U.S. Department of Health and Human Services
healthit.gov/patients-families
202-690-7151
onc.request@hhs.gov
includes information on electronic health records and other e-patient advocacy issues

Regina Holliday's Medical Advocacy Blog
reginaholliday.blogspot.com

U.S. Department of Health & Human Services
Office for Civil Rights
"Health Information Privacy"
hhs.gov/ocr/privacy/hipaa/understanding/consumers
How to File a Complaint
hhs.gov/ocr/privacy/hipaa/complaints/index.html
Regional offices directory
hhs.gov/ocr/office/about/rgn-hqaddresses.html

Clinical Trials

Center for Clinical Trials Education
lupusfoundation.org/clinicaltrials

Lupus Trials
lupustrials.org

Acknowledgments

This book is a culmination of much of what I learned from people with lupus and their loved ones, and from colleagues and health care professionals in the lupus community. Thank you for sharing your stories, knowledge, and wisdom that are, in turn, gifts to others.

Thank you to Demos Health Publishing for asking me to write this and giving me the opportunity to share this information, and to Lee Oglesby for initially reaching out to me. Norman Graubart and Michael O'Connor, I appreciate your editorial experise and support, and kindness. A special thanks to executive editor, Julia Pastore, who guided and supported me through the entire process. You are a talented editor with much compassion and patience. I am exceptionally lucky to have been paired with you.

Dr. Anca Askanase, lupus expert and rheumatologist, you already do so much for the lupus community, yet you found time to review a chapter for me and answer my questions. I am grateful for this, for your constant cheerleading, and your dedication to your patients.

Diane Gross, who I first went to when I learned about this opportunity, thank you for your continued support, the opportunities you have given me, and your intelligence and mentorship that have helped me grow exponentially.

Margy Meislin, I am grateful for the space you always give me to think things through and for your gentle personal and professional guidance and support both with this book and writing, in general.

Amy Caron, thank you for your supportiveness and helpfulness; I was relieved that, despite your deadlines, you took the time to answer my questions and share your expertise with me.

Kathleen A. Arntsen, I deeply appreciate the time you took to read through the book and the kind words you shared, but also all that you have done for nearly 30 years for lupus, chronic illness, and patient advocacy. Your importance to these communities cannot be understated. Thanks for all that you do!

Elyse Reyes, I am glad to be able to turn to you for your unique perspective and sharp critical thinking skills. Thank you for your feedback, willingness, and kindness.

Jennifer Faylor, thank you for reaching out to me when I needed the assistance, and for connecting me with Nigina Khasidova.

Nigina, you barely knew me, but you took the time to provide me with excellent help. Thank you.

Thank you Jenna Valente (of Jenna Karin Photography), best friend and photographer, not only for the head shot for this book, but for your love and support for this project and our profound friendship.

John Joseph Cina, you, my life partner who selflessly prioritizes my endeavors, I am especially grateful for your constant listening, loving encouragement, and celebration of my achievements.

And thank you to my parents, Luz and Asghar Rowshandel, and my sisters, Allyson Rowshandel and Caroline Reddy, for your love, pride and excitement, and always believing in my ability to write.

Index

acupuncture, 28
acute cutaneous lupus erythematosus
    (ACLE), 5
ADA compliance, 98, 114
advance directives, 93–95
advocacy
    creating lupus awareness, 115–117
    educating doctors, 116
    for health care policies and
        funding, 117
    online, 116
    and patient-centered medicine, 118–119
alcohol, 50, 108
alternative treatments, 28–29. *See also*
    treatments
antinuclear antibody (ANA) test, 8
aromatherapy, 28
arthritis, 7
autoimmune disease, 3–5, 8, 112

birth control, 85. *See also* family
    planning
body pain, 6, 7, 8, 28
breathing exercises, 63

cardiologists, 12
central nervous system, 7
children
    addressing concerns, 89
    balancing chores, 90
    behavioral changes in, 88
    explaining lupus to, 87–88
    help with, 90
    quality time with, 89
chronic cutaneous lupus
    erythematosus (CCLE), 5

clinical trials, 119
clinics, 15
college, 107–110
    advocacy and support, 110
    course load during, 108–109
    disability and health services, 108
    study and attendance concerns, 109, 107
complementary treatments, 28.
    See also treatments
concentration difficulties, 8. *See also*
    lupus fog
creativity, 59
cutaneous lupus
    erythematosus (CLE), 5

daily tasks, 54, 61–62
dating, 79–80
depression, 42–43
diagnosis of lupus, 6–7
dietary tips, 47–49
disability benefits
    appealing a denial, 105
    application paperwork, 103–104
    date of disability, 104–105
    exclusions, 105
    expedited reinstatement, 106
    financial planning and, 101–102
    Freelancers and, 105
    legal help with, 102, 103
    long-term disability, 101, 103
    short-term disability, 101
    Social Security benefits and, 102
    support from doctors, 104
    work history, 104
discoid lupus erythematosus (DLE), 5
discoid rash, 7
doctor-hopping, 21

doctor of osteopathic medicine (DO), 6
doctor visits, 17–21
doctors, finding, 6, 9–11, 21. *See also*
     rheumatologist
doctors, helping, 116
drug-induced lupus, 5–6
drug interactions, 23–24. *See also*
     medications

e-patients, 118
education, 11, 107–110, 115–116
elimination diet, 49. *See also*
     nutritional tips
emergency grants, 16
emergency plans, 113
emergency rooms, 15
emotional crisis, 43
emotional distress, 5, 43, 65–67
employment concerns. *See also*
     disability benefits
  employment alternatives, 99
  flares and, 98
  health priorities, 97
  informing employer, 97
  planning ahead for, 100
  requesting time off, 98
  stopping work, 99
  stress and, 55
  vocational rehabilitation, 106
  work environment, 98
  working from home, 99
  workplace accommodations, 98–99
energy levels, 56–57
exercise
  as complementary treatment, 28
  benefits of, 50
  breathing exercises, 63
  concerns about, 28
  modifying, 28, 50
  tips for, 50
external concerns
  hair loss, 8, 65–67
  makeup tips, 67–68
  self-conscious feelings, 65–67
  skin protection, 50, 67–68
  weight fluctuations, 68

family
  communicating with, 72–73
  holidays with, 76–77
  social life with, 75–76
  support for, 74
  support from, 43, 54–56,
     71–77
family planning
  birth control pills, 85
  breastfeeding concerns, 85
  flares and, 84
  medications and, 83
  postbirthing monitoring, 85
  pregnancy, 84
fatigue
  dating and, 80
  describing, 73, 81–82
  diagnosing, 8
  energy levels and, 56
fevers, 8
fibromyalgia, 8
financial needs, 97
financial planning, 101–102
flares
  doctor visits for, 17–19
  explanation of, 3
  family planning and, 84
  planning ahead for, 53–55, 90
  self-care during, 55
  stress and, 53–56
  work and, 98
food journal, 49
foods
  allergies from, 48–49
  dietary tips, 47–49
  holiday meals, 76
  nutritional foods, 47–49
  processed foods, 48
  sensitivity to, 48–49
  tracking meals, 49
forgetfulness, 8. *See also* lupus fog
forgiveness, 57
friends
  communicating with, 72–73
  holidays with, 76–77
  social life with, 75–76

friends (*cont.*)
  support for, 74
  support from, 39, 43, 54–56, 71–77
funding issues, 117

grants, 16
gratitude, 19, 58
grief, 41–42

hair loss, 8, 65–67
health care advocate, 117
health care centers, 15
health care
  communicating wishes for, 93–94
  doctors for, 6, 9–11, 21
  end-of-life care, 94
  legal help with, 95
  power of attorney, 95
  specialists, 12–13, 40–41
  wills, 93, 94, 95
health care funding, 117
health care policies, 117
health care professionals
  appreciation for, 21
  attributes of, 18
  cardiologists, 12
  communicating with, 11–13,
    19–21
  education of, 11
  finding, 6, 9–11, 21
  nephrologists, 12
  neurologists, 12
  rheumatologists, 6–13
  second opinions from, 13
  specialists, 12–13, 40–41
  visits to, 17–21
health care wishes, 93–95
health department assistance, 15
health insurance
  charity care options, 14
  COBRA, 14
  during travel, 113
  level of, 13
  low-cost clinics, 15
  network referrals, 10

  obtaining coverage, 14
  underinsured and uninsured, 13–15
health risks, 47
healthy lifestyle
  maintaining, 47–51
  nutrition for, 47–49
  striving for, 49–51
  tips for, 47–51
heart issues, 7
hematologic disorder, 7–8
herbs, 29–31
higher education, 107–110. *See also* college
holidays, 76–77
hospitals
  charity care options, 14
  community clinics, 15
  doctors in, 10
  non-profit hospitals, 15
  rheumatology departments in, 10
household concerns, 54, 61–62

"I" statements, 20, 71
immune system disorder, 3–5, 8, 112
infertility concerns, 83
inflammation, 7
information, remembering, 61–63
information, sharing, 115–119
insurance, 10, 13–15, 113. *See also* health
  insurance

joint pain, 8

kidney problems, 7

laughter, 60
legal matters, 93–95, 102–103
limitations, 56, 72. *See also* support
lung issues, 7
lupus
  advocacy, 115–117, 118
  cause of, 4
  chronic conditions, 4

lupus (*cont.*)
  describing to others, 73, 79–80,
    87–88, 109–110, 113
  development of, 4
  diagnosis of, 6–7
  differences in, 40
  as "Great Imitator," 6
  medical care for, 9–21
  medications for, 23–27
  men with, 45–46
  personal appearance and, 65–68
  symptoms of, 6–8
  treatments for, 4, 27–32
  types of, 3, 5–6
  understanding, 3–8
lupus advocacy, 115–117, 118.
lupus fog
  consistency, 63
  daily tasks, 61–62
  decluttering tips, 62
  explanation of, 8
  log for, 64
  managing, 61–64
  note-taking tips, 61–62
  picture-taking tips, 62
  recording experiences of, 64
  remembering information, 61–63
lupus organizations
  finding, 9–10
  for insurance assistance, 15
  involvement in, 115–116

malar rash, 7
massage therapy, 28
medical care
  during college, 107
  doctors for, 6, 9–11, 21
  obtaining, 9–21
  specialists for, 12–13, 40–41
  during travel, 112–113
medical history, 6, 17
medical identification jewelry, 26,
    53–54
medical information, organizing, 53–56
medical paperwork, 103–104

medications, 23–27. *See also*
    treatments
  clinical trials, 119
  dosing instructions, 25
  food and drug interactions,
    23–24
  identification jewelry for, 26,
    53–54
  infertility concerns, 83
  keeping list of, 25, 53–54
  managing, 23–27
  mood changes and, 73
  organizing, 24
  and original bottles, 24, 114
  reminders for, 24–25
  side effects of, 23, 25–27, 26–27
  stopping, 25, 29
  traveling and, 24, 111–112, 114
  understanding, 23
meditation, 58
memory issues, 61–63. *See also*
    lupus fog
men with lupus, 45–46
mindfulness, 58
mood changes, 73
mouth ulcers, 7
muscle pain, 8, 23, 28
musculoskeletal conditions, 6, 8

neonatal lupus, 5
nephrologists, 12
neurological symptoms, 7
neurologists, 12
nonerosive arthritis, 7
nose ulcers, 7
note-taking tips, 20, 61–63
nutritional tips
  dietary tips, 47–49
  food allergies, 48–49
  holiday meals, 76
  tracking meals, 49

occupational therapy, 28
organization tips

organization tips (*cont.*)
  for daily tasks, 54, 61–62
  decluttering tips, 62
  for lupus fog, 62–63
  for medical information, 53–56
  for medications, 24
  to-do lists, 63
organizations
  finding, 9–10
  for insurance assistance, 15
  involvement in, 115–116

pain. *See also* treatments
  body pain, 6, 7, 8, 28
  chest pain, 7
  describing, 20, 73, 82
  and exercise, 50
  nonerosive arthritis, 7
  and poor sleep, 50–51
  Raynaud's phenomenon, 8, 82
  relieving, 23, 28, 58, 60, 82
  and sex, 81–82
  specifics about, 73
parenting tips
  addressing concerns, 89
  canceling plans, 88
  for chores, 90
  communication tips, 89
  explaining lupus, 87–88
  making promises, 88
  observing behaviors, 88
  parenting support group, 89
  planning for flares, 90
  quality time, 89
  for self-care, 90
participatory medicine, 118–119
passions, 60
patient-centered medicine, 118–119
personal appearance
  concerns about, 65–68
  hair loss, 8, 65–67
  makeup tips, 67–68
  self-conscious feelings, 65–67
  skin protection, 50, 67–68
  weight fluctuations, 68

pharmaceutical companies, 16
pharmacies, 16–17
photosensitivity, 7
physical needs, 97
physical therapy, 28
positive antinuclear antibody (ANA)
    test, 8
pre-existing conditions, 105
pregnancy, 84. *See also* family planning
prescriptions
  assistance with, 16–17
  cost-comparisons of, 16–17
  discount card for, 18
primary care physician, 10
pseudoscience, 32–35
psychological distress, 5
psychosis, 7
psychotherapists, 40–41

rashes, 7
Raynaud's phenomenon, 8, 82
rejection, handling, 80
relationships
  balance in, 80–81
  dating, 79–80
  describing lupus, 79–80
  with family and friends, 71–77
  family planning, 83–85
  fatigue and, 80
  finding the right person, 80
  honesty in, 80–81
  including partner, 81
  parenting tips, 87–90
  rejection in, 80
  romantic relationships,
      79–85
  sexual relationships, 81–83
religion, 58
renal problems, 7
resources, 123–132
rest, 57, 109, 114
retina toxicity, 26
retirement, 102
rheumatic diseases, 6
rheumatoid arthritis, 7

rheumatologist
    appreciation for, 21
    attributes of, 18
    communicating with, 11–13, 19–21
    deal breakers, 20
    definition of, 6
    finding, 6, 9–11, 21
    reputation of, 12
    researching, 11–12
    second opinions from, 13
    selecting, 6, 11–12
    support during visits, 20
    visits to, 17–21

saying "no," 56
science, fake, 32–35
science, real, 32
second opinions, 13
seizures, 7
self-advocacy, 19
self-care, 55, 81, 90, 108, 110
self-conscious feelings, 65
self-employment, 105
self-forgiveness, 57
sexual relationships, 81–83
    erectile dysfunction, 82
    family planning, 83–85
    fatigue and, 82
    gynecological problems, 82
    low sex drive, 81
    pain and, 82
    vaginal dryness, 82
Sjögren's syndrome, 6, 8
skin lupus, 5
sleep requirements, 51
sleep, tracking, 51
smoking, 49–50
social life. See also relationships
    dating, 79–80
    with family, 71–77
    with friends, 75–76
    maintaining, 75–76
Social Security Disability Insurance
    (SSDI), 102, 103
specialists, 12–13, 40–41

spirituality, 58
stress
    bill-paying concerns, 54
    breaks from, 59
    energy levels and, 56–57
    flares and, 53–56
    holidays and, 76
    household concerns, 54
    managing, 53–60
    meditation for, 58
    reducing, 58–60
    rest and, 57
    support for, 54–56
    time-management skills, 57
    work concerns, 55
subacute cutaneous lupus
    erythematosus (SCLE), 5
suicidal concerns, 43
sunscreen, 50, 67-68
Supplemental Security Income (SSI),
    102, 103
supplements/herbs, 29–31
support
    during college, 110
    during doctor visits, 20
    from family, 43, 54–56, 71–77
    finding, 10, 39–41
    from friends, 39, 43, 54–56, 71–77
    groups for, 10, 39–40, 72, 89, 110, 117
    lack of, 74
    for men, 45–46
    for parents, 89
    for stressful times, 54–56
symptoms of lupus, 6–8
systemic lupus erythematosus (SLE),
    3–4. See also lupus

tai chi, 28
time-management skills, 57
to-do lists, 63
traveling
    with autoimmune disease, 112
    comfort concerns, 114
    describing lupus to others, 113
    discussing with doctor, 111

traveling (*cont.*)
  emergencies during, 113
  flying concerns, 114
  health insurance concerns, 113
  hotel concerns, 114
  insurance for, 112
  medical care concerns, 112–113
  medications and, 111–112
  packing medications, 111–112
  planning ahead for, 113
  rest during, 114
  vaccinations and, 112
treatments. *See also* medications
  alternative treatments, 28–29
  checking the research, 29–30
  complementary treatments, 28
  exercise and, 28
  improvements in, 4
  vitamins and supplements, 30–31

ulcers, 7

vaccinations, 112
vision problems, 26
vitamins, 30–31
vocational rehabilitation
      programs, 106
volunteerism, 60

water aerobics, 28
weight fluctuations, 68
wills, 93, 94, 95
work concerns. *See* employment
      concerns; disability benefits

yoga, 28

About the Author

Jessica Rowshandel, LMSW, is a social worker and the former Director of Social Services of the S.L.E. Lupus Foundation in New York City. She was the author of the Foundation's monthly column about coping with lupus, called *Jessica's Coping with Lupus Corner*. She facilitated lupus support groups and provided counseling for people with lupus and their loved ones. She also created a photovoice program for people with lupus to learn to use photography to express what it means to live with the disease. Her interest in photovoice developed from her personal interests in coping with chronic illness, social justice, and the arts. She obtained her master's degree in social work from Columbia University and her bachelor's degree in forensic psychology from John Jay College of Criminal Justice. She was born in New York City to Iranian and Puerto Rican parents and now lives in California.